Mayada JEMAA
Khouloud ATTI

Nanoparticle Technology in Endodontics

Mayada JEMAA
Khouloud ATTI

Nanoparticle Technology in Endodontics

ScienciaScripts

Cover image: www.ingimage.com

This book is a translation from the original published under ISBN 978-620-6-71300-5.

Publisher:
Sciencia Scripts
is a trademark of
Dodo Books Indian Ocean Ltd. and OmniScriptum S.R.L publishing group

120 High Road, East Finchley, London, N2 9ED, United Kingdom
Str. Armeneasca 28/1, office 1, Chisinau MD-2012, Republic of Moldova, Europe
Printed at: see last page
ISBN: 978-620-8-26806-0

CONTENTS

INTRODUCTION..2

CLASSIFICATIONS 3

THE NANOPARTICLES MOST COMMONLY USED IN ENDODONTICS 5

CONCLUSION..40

REFERENCES 41

INTRODUCTION

Endodontics is a branch of dentistry that focuses on the pulp organ and periapical tissues. The oral cavity is constantly exposed to a multitude of micro-organisms. present in dental plaque. Dental biofilm bacteria can form a complex community that protects pathogenic micro-organisms, antimicrobial agents and evades host defence mechanisms. Although significant progress has been made in endodontic techniques, certain challenges remain, notably the effective eradication of persistent infections and the hermetic obturation of the root canal system. Infections can also spread from other areas of the body via the bloodstream. The success of endodontic treatment depends on the complete elimination of bacteria and damaged canal tissue. However, clinical studies have shown that bacteria persist despite the use of effective antimicrobial agents. The complex anatomy of the root canal system may allow bacteria to localise in areas inaccessible to antimicrobial agents. In addition, the efficacy of antibacterial agents may be limited by factors such as the concentration, time and volume used in root canals.Over the years, endodontics has benefited from significant advances in the materials and techniques used for treatment. Nanotechnology has been defined by the National Nanotechnology Initiative,(154) as the creation of materials, devices or functional systems by controlling nanoparticles. These measure between 1 and 100 nanometres (nm) and have attracted growing interest as key components in endodontics. Because of their small size, nanoparticles (NPs) have a large surface area per unit mass, giving them unique properties and enhanced performance compared with their larger-scale counterparts. They may be more chemically reactive, have different melting or boiling points, exhibit improved electrical or thermal conductivity, and may even have different optical properties.These nanometric particles may represent a new strategy for the treatment and prevention of dental infections. Their applications in endodontics are vast and varied. They include improving the properties of the restorative materials used, modulating antimicrobial properties to combat persistent bacterial infections and promoting tissue regeneration to restore the vitality of the dental pulp. The aim of our work is firstly to define nanotechnology and take stock of the nanoparticles most commonly used in endodontics. Secondly, we will describe the various clinical applications of nanoparticles in endodontics.

CLASSIFICATIONS

Because of their extremely small size, nanoparticles have a wide range of properties and applications. To better understand and categorise these nanoparticles, various classification criteria have been established. Among these criteria, structural configuration emerges as one of the most relevant. Depending on their structural configuration, nanoparticles can be grouped into three main categories: organic nanoparticles, inorganic nanoparticles, carbon-based nanoparticles and composite nanoparticles. (74)

1- Organic nanoparticles [(75)]

As their name suggests, they are made up of organic substances such as proteins, polymers, lipids, carbohydrates, etc. Some of the best-known examples are liposomes, dendrimers, micelles and ferritin. Among the best-known examples are liposomes, dendrimers, micelles and ferritin (Fig.1). They are generally non-toxic, biodegradable and have non-covalent intermolecular interactions that are often unstable. In addition, the development of biodegradable organic nanoparticles, which alleviate the toxicity problems associated with the use of metallic nanoparticles, is arousing genuine interest, leading to their rapid use in the biomedical and pharmaceutical fields.

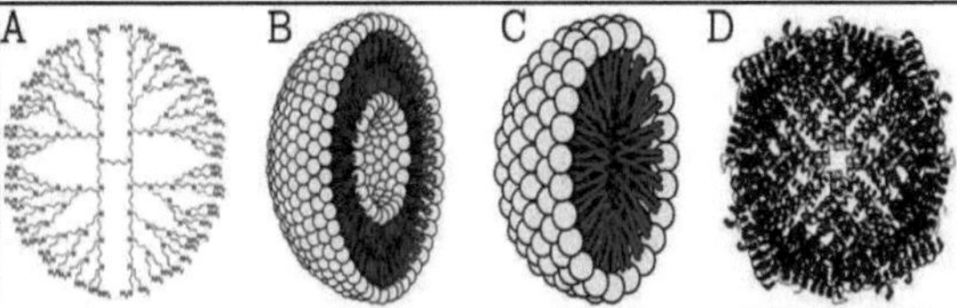

Figure 1: Organic nanoparticles: (A) Dendrimers;(B) Micelles;(C) Liposomes and (D) Ferritin.[(75)]

2- Carbon-based nanoparticles [(75)]

The nanoparticles in this category are made exclusively of carbon. Due to their unique physicochemical properties at the nanoscale (high electrical conductivity, electronic affinity, high resistance, thermal and optical properties) and the distinctive characteristics of hybridised carbon sp2-bonds, carbon-based nanoparticles have a wide range of applications in drug delivery, bio-imaging and monitoring microbial ecology. Examples include fullerenes, graphene, carbon nanotubes, carbon nanofibres and carbon black (Fig.2).

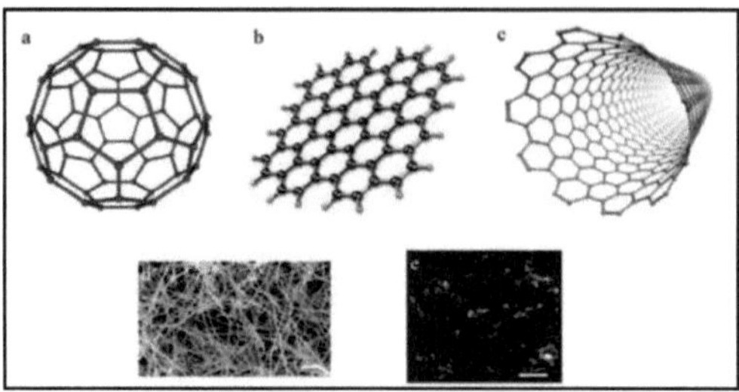

Figure 2: Carbon-based nanoparticles: (A) fullerenes; (B) graphene; (C) carbon nanotubes; (d) carbon nanofibres and (e) carbon black.(16)

3- **Inorganic nanoparticles**

Inorganic nanoparticles are attracting growing interest because they offer dazzling properties such as non-toxicity, biocompatibility, hydrophilicity and significant stability compared with organic materials. (16) This class includes :

▪ **Metallic nanoparticles** (16)**:** these are known for their distinctive characteristics such as a high surface/volume ratio, the pore size, surface charge and surface charge density, crystalline and amorphous structures, shapes such as spherical and cylindrical and colour, reactivity and sensitivity to environmental factors such as air, humidity, heat and sunlight, etc. The most commonly used examples are: gold (Au), silver (Ag), zinc (Zn), cobalt (Co), copper (Cu), aluminium (Al), cadmium (Cd), iron (Fe), and lead (Pb).

▪ **Metal oxide nanoparticles** (16)**:** They are synthesised from their respective metal nanoparticles, by an oxidation reaction, in order to increase their reactivity and efficiency.

▪ **Semiconductor nanoparticles** (67)**:** These are characterised by properties between metals and non-metals. From a structural point of view, these semiconductor nanoparticles have large band gaps, which are responsible for a significant change in their properties as the band gap is adjusted.

▪ **Ceramic nanoparticles** (129)**:** These are inorganic structures mainly formed by carbonates, carbides, phosphates and oxides of metals and metalloids, such as titanium and calcium. They are mainly used in biomedical applications because of their high stability and loading capacity.

4- **Composite nanoparticles**

They are combinations of nanoparticles with other nanoparticles or nanoparticles combined with larger materials or more complex structures. Consequently, they are multiphase nanomaterials with one phase on the nanometric scale (74).

THE NANOPARTICLES MOST COMMONLY USED IN ENDODONTICS

1- Chitosan

1-1- Definition [7]

Chitosan (CS) is an organic, polycationic compound and polymer that is very abundant in nature, with a specific structure and properties. This biopolymer is a deacetylated derivative of chitin, obtained commercially from shrimps and crabs (an N-acetylglucosamine polymer) by 2-4 alkaline deacetylation (Na OH, 40-50%).Being a cationic polysaccharide, under neutral or basic pH conditions chitosan contains free amino groups and is therefore insoluble in water. Aqueous solutions of 1-3% acetic acid are usually used to solubilise CS. (114)

1-2- Properties

Chitosan nanoparticles (CS-NP) are biocompatible with living tissue, since they do not cause allergic reactions or rejection. In fact, they break down slowly into harmless products (amino sugars), which are completely absorbed by the human body. They break down under the action of ferments. They are therefore non-toxic and are easily eliminated from the body without causing any concomitant secondary reactions. (7) The structure of chitosan is similar to the components of the extracellular matrix and is therefore used to reinforce collagen constructs. For example, in general medicine, it is useful as a dressing that mimics the native extracellular matrix, ensuring the appropriate microenvironment of the wound, thereby accelerating healing. These nanoparticles are known for their excellent antibacterial, antiviral and antifungal properties. When attacking bacteria, gram-positive bacteria were more sensitive than gram-negative ones, while gram-negative bacteria were less sensitive. Minimum inhibitory concentrations (MICs) varied from 18 to 5000 ppm depending on the organism, pH, molecular weight, chemical modifications, the presence of lipids and proteins, and above all the degree of deacetylation (DD), which is known to influence antibacterial activity. The higher the DD, the greater the number of amino groups per unit of glucosamine and, consequently, the greater the antibacterial efficacy of chitosan. (122) In addition, chitosan nanoparticles can offer good adhesion, coagulation and immunostimulation capacity. (32)

2- Graphene and its derivatives

2-1- Definition

Graphene (G), the thinnest and strongest element known, is one of the crystalline forms of carbon. It is a two-dimensional atomic sheet, less than 10 nm thick, composed of sp2-hybridised carbon atoms arranged in a honeycomb lattice. It was successfully isolated by Geim and Kostya for the first time in 2004. (61, 90) Graphene has two main derivatives, namely graphene oxide (GO) and reduced graphene oxide (rGO). GO can be obtained by oxidation of graphite and rGO can be synthesised by reduction of GO. (127)

2-2- Properties

2-2-1- Biocompatibility

Graphene and its derivatives have attracted a great deal of interest in the fields of biomedicine and dentistry. Consequently, their cytotoxicity has been systematically examined prior to their clinical application. The biological toxicity of graphene nanoparticle (G-NP) based nanomaterials on various cell lines, including fibroblasts, epithelial cells and neuronal cells, has been evaluated. It is described by common mechanisms including the production of reactive oxygen species (ROS), cell membrane damage and alterations in the expression of apoptosis-related genes. The results of in vitro and in vivo studies have shown that the cytotoxicity of graphene and its derivatives is influenced by several factors, such as their concentration, shape, size, dispersibility and functional surface. (149) The oral biocompatibility of some graphene-based nanomaterials, mainly graphene oxide, reduced graphene oxide, polymethyl methacrylate (PMMA) resin loaded with graphene-silver nanoparticles (G-AgNP), and incorporated sodium alginate assemblies (GOSA/rGOSA), was studied. The weakest cytotoxic effect on human dental follicle stem cells (hDFSCs) was observed with GO by inducing oxidative stress without damaging the cell membrane. Concerning nitrogen-doped graphene, the good safety profile is at a concentration of 4 μg/mL, and if a concentration of (40 μg/mL) is exceeded, there will be a reduction in cell viability and damage to the membrane by mechanical effects. (90)In contrast, G-AgNP-loaded PMMA resin was able to decrease the viability of dysplastic oral keratinocytes and dental pulp stem cells (DPSC), but cell viability remained greater than 75% compared to controls. Another study by Dreanca et al. 2020(51) assessed the biocompatibility of two graphene-based dental composite materials, a cement and a light-curing hybrid restorative composite. The results 7 weeks after implantation of these materials in a mandibular defect, showed the absence of significant in vitro cytotoxicity on hDFSCs and dysplastic oral keratinocytes, and the absence of in vivo symptoms of acute toxicity or local inflammation in the animals. This demonstrates the good biocompatibility of graphene-based dental composites (90) Generally speaking, the majority of studies have shown that graphene and its derivatives are biocompatible materials that can also be used in tissue engineering. (65)

2-2-2- Antimicrobial activity

In addition to biocompatibility, antimicrobial efficacy against oral pathogens is essential to the success of biomaterials. Graphene-based nanomaterials and its derivatives have antibacterial activity against Gram-positive and Gram-negative bacteria and are bactericidal against the majority of dental pathogenic microorganisms. A study conducted by Liu et al. 2011, (91) compared the antimicrobial efficacy of graphite, graphite oxide, GO and rGO as a function of time and concentration when exposed to Escherichia coli (E. coli). The results of this study showed that GO exhibited the highest antibacterial activity, with 69.3% inactivation of bacterial cells, compared with graphite, graphite oxide and rGO, which showed inactivation rates of 26.1%, 15% and 45.9% respectively. Most of these bactericidal properties appeared during the first four hours of interaction with these graphene derivatives. The induction of oxidative stress has been suggested as a key process in the antibacterial mechanism (109).

Research carried out by Chen J et al. in 2020(42) revealed that the addition of 2% by reduced weight of graphene-silver nanoparticles in glass ions caused a significant reduction in the number of Streptococcus mutans (S. mutans). The findings of this study validated the efficacy of graphene-based nanomaterials and its derivatives for direct inhibition of bacteria, while also indirectly contributing to improving the antibacterial properties of metallic nanomaterials, in particular zinc oxide (ZnO), silver and copper nanoparticles. GO can also be combined with new technologies to obtain its antibacterial activity against S. mutans by delivering nucleic acids and photosensitisers. (90) (Fig.3 (A))

However, G-NPs have antibacterial activity in a dose-dependent manner. In fact, at high concentrations, GO inhibits the formation of biofilms of Gram-positive and Gram-negative bacteria, and at low concentrations, GO can promote their formation, creating a reaction completely opposite to the intention. For a concentration of less than 50 µg/ml of GO in a nutrient medium solution, not only was there an absence of antimicrobial activity, but GO also promoted bacterial growth by acting as a biofilm itself (127).

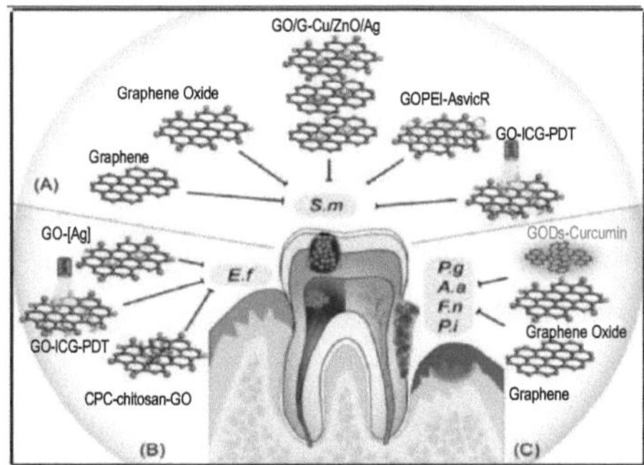

Figure 3: Antibacterial action of graphene nanoparticles and its derivatives on oral bacteria(90).
Inhibition of cariogenic bacteria :
Control of dental pulp infection.
Suppression of periodontal pathogens.

2-2-3- Other properties [82]

The origin of graphene's extraordinary properties lies in its unique honeycomb structure. Each carbon atom in graphene is linked to three neighbouring atoms by covalent bonds. This gives it exceptional structural rigidity, which contributes to its formidable mechanical properties, with a Young's modulus of 1 TPa, a tensile strength of 130 GPa and a modulus of elasticity of 32 GPa. However, a carbon atom has four bonds, whereas in graphene, each atom contributes an unbound electron, which is free to move through the crystal, resulting in excellent electrical conductivity. Graphene also has superior thermal conductivity (5300 Wm-1K) and ultra-high electron mobility (250,000 cm^2 /Vs) at room temperature. Exceptional carrier transport speed (up to 40 GHz), current transport (high up to 109A/cm^2), maximum specific surface area (2630 m^2 g-1) and magnificent optical properties are also remarkable. (82)

3- The money

3-1- Definition

Metal nanoparticles are known for their unique physicochemical properties. They have a specific surface area, a high fraction of surface atoms and remarkable optical, electronic, antibacterial and magnetic properties.Silver nanoparticles (AgNPs) are the most fascinating of the metallic nanoparticles involved in biomedical applications. Silver nanoparticles or nanosilver is a metallic material based on silver atoms whose size is generally between 1 and 100 nm. As with the synthesis of metallic nanoparticles, various physical, chemical and biological methods have been adopted for the synthesis of silver nanoparticles (103). The chemical approach, most frequently used in dentistry, is based on the chemical reduction of silver nanoparticles. In the physical approach, AgNP synthesis methods are essentially based on evaporation-condensation and laser ablation. However, biological synthesis or "green chemistry" is a rapidly developing method used in the development of silver nanoparticles. Prokaryotic organisms, such as bacteria, and eukaryotic organisms, such as fungi and plants, are used as potential biological reducers for the reduction of metal ions. This technique appears to be a sustainable alternative for making the synthesis process more environmentally friendly, less complicated and less costly than chemical and physical methods.Biocompatibility is a key advantage of this technique, especially in biotechnological applications, particularly in the medical, pharmacological and biological fields. In dentistry, the organisms commonly used to synthesise silver nanoparticles are plants. (1, 103)

3-2- Properties

3-2-1- Biocompatibility

The application of silver nanoparticles in the oral cavity, to combat infectious diseases and microbes, requires in vitro and in vivo explorations to examine the undesirable effects of these products, and also to meet safety and biocompatibility requirements. Moreover, toxicity is always correlated with the dose administered and the duration of contact. Consideration of direct contact with the oral cavity, teeth and surrounding tissues is of crucial importance because of the potentially harmful effects of silver nanoparticle treatment in the context of endodontic applications. (25) As irrigation agents, silver nanoparticles at a concentration of 50 μg/ml (0.005%) have demonstrated antibacterial properties, while concentrations exceeding 80 μg/ml could be considered cytotoxic. Studies conducted by Frankova et al. in 2016,(57) indicated that silver nanoparticles with a spherical structure, with an average size of 10 nm, are likely to be biocompatible with keratinocytes and fibroblasts.(25)

3-2-2- Antimicrobial activity

Among metallic nanoparticles, silver nanoparticles are of particular interest in research, due to their antimicrobial potential and their biological activity against bacteria, fungi and enveloped viruses.The biological characteristics of silver, in particular its antibacterial activity, have given this element a significant reputation in dentistry. Indeed, AgNPs have demonstrated broad-spectrum antibacterial action, targeting both Gram-positive and Gram-negative bacteria, as well as various drug-resistant strains. (25)

It is relevant to note that the antibacterial properties of silver are primarily attributable to the rates of silver ion (Ag+) release. This release of Ag+ ions is more pronounced when fine silver nanoparticles (particle size < 10 nm) are used than when larger ones are used, resulting in increased antibacterial efficacy. (25)Overall, silver ions disrupt ATP molecules, interfere with DNA replication, trigger the formation of ROS and cause direct damage to the cell membrane, leading to the rupture of internal cell organelles and, ultimately, bacterial death.

AgNPs also have an antibacterial action against Gram-negative bacteria by creating pits in the cell wall. As a result, a membrane with this morphology shows a significant increase in permeability, leading to cell death (25). In line with the findings of Holla et al. in 2012, (93)a minimum inhibitory concentration of 0.04 mg/ml of AgNPs effectively inhibits Streptococcus mutans.In addition, Chávez-Andrade et al. in 2019(41) analysed the antimicrobial and anti-adhesive properties of silver nanoparticles coated with polyvinyl alcohol and farnesol against Entérococcus faecalis (E.faecalis), Candida albicans (C.albicans) and Pseudomonas aeruginosa (P.aeruginosa). The results of these investigations demonstrated the efficacy of AgNPs as an adjuvant to endodontic treatment, both for root canal disinfection and for the inhibition of biofilm formation (146).

Silver nanoparticles were initially studied for their antimicrobial potential against bacteria. However, they have also been shown to be effective against various types of virus, including human immunodeficiency virus (HIV), hepatitis B virus, herpes simplex virus type 1, respiratory syncytial virus (RSV), influenza virus, Tacaribe virus and monkey pox virus (59).

AgNPs have been suggested to promote wound healing due to their potential biological properties (antibacterial properties, antioxidant properties, anti-inflammatory effects). AgNPs are compatible with fibroblasts and keratinocytes, demonstrating an ability to inhibit the production of pro-inflammatory cytokines such as IL-6, IL-1 beta and tumour necrosis factor (TNF)-alpha (4). Finally, we'll look at the antifungal activity of silver nanoparticles, which was evaluated by Keuk-Jun Kim et al. in 2008.(80) The results showed that AgNPs exhibited antifungal effects. on the fungi tested, while showing limited haemolytic effects on human erythrocytes(80).

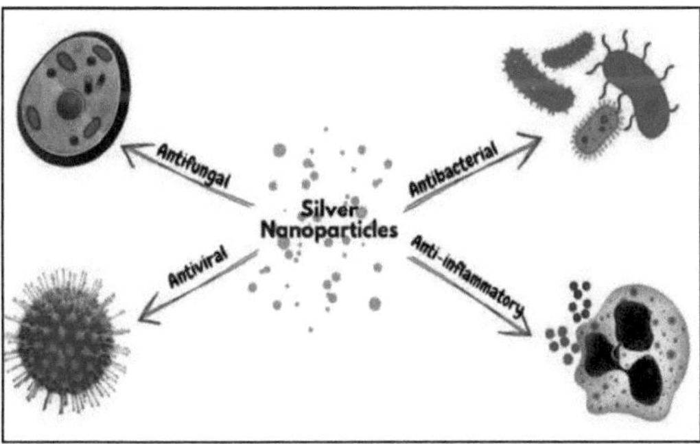

Figure 4: Biological properties of silver nanoparticles(4)

3-2-3- Other properties [117]

By virtue of their small size and large surface area, these silver nanoparticles exhibit excellent electrical, optical and thermal properties. They have excellent electrical conductivity and are remarkably malleable and ductile. These silver nanoparticles are also used as an alternative radiopacifying agent to impart the required radiopacity to calcium silicate cements (CSC) and to assess the purity of radiopacifying agents.

4- Metal oxides

4-1- Definition

By definition, metal oxides are composed of oxide anions and metal cations. In reality, oxides represent the "natural" form of metals in their native state, to which they tend to return "spontaneously". (155)

The variability of the electronic structure of metal oxide nanoparticles (MeO-NP) gives them unique physicochemical properties, making them capable of interacting in a distinctive way with biological systems. (115)

Zinc oxide nanoparticles (ZnO-NP) have been extensively investigated in the field of endodontics compared to other metal oxide nanoparticles, due to their biological properties as antimicrobial agents.

ZnO is an n-type semiconducting metal oxide. (62) Its crystalline surface has a number of defects and interstitial sites (Fig.5), which are responsible for its versatile properties such as mechanical, thermal, electrical and optical properties. (83)

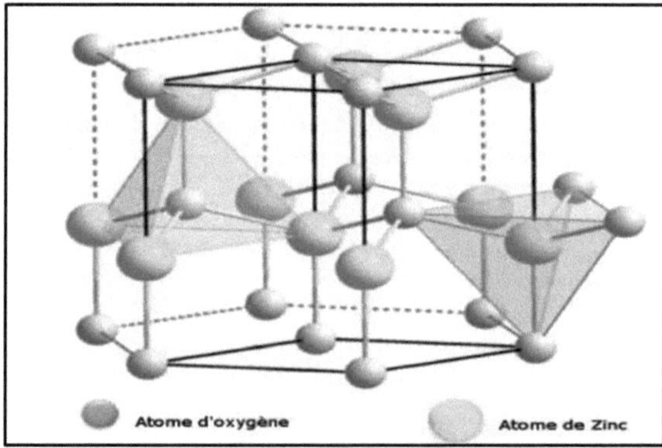

Figure 5: Crystal structure of ZnO(78)

4-2- Properties

4-2-1- Biocompatibility

Metal oxide nanoparticles exhibit a wide range of toxicities, which depend on the specific nature of the metal oxide used, as well as its modifiable intrinsic parameters. The toxicity of certain metal oxide nanoparticles can vary depending on the dose, the duration of exposure, and the cell and tissue types involved. This toxic phenomenon is mainly attributable to the pro-oxidant nature of metal oxide nanoparticles. It has been suggested that metal oxide nanoparticles may induce increased toxicity compared with their micrometric particle counterparts, due to their reduced dimensions and large surface areas. (62)A study conducted by Johanna Gustafsson et al. in 2009(77) assessed the toxicity of various metal oxide nanoparticles on A549 cells, a human alveolar epithelial cell line. The results indicated that copper nanoparticles (CuO-NP) showed more pronounced cytotoxicity and genotoxicity than several other metal oxide particles examined, while iron oxide nanoparticles (Fe-NP) showed less toxicity. However, it was observed that these nanoparticles showed a significantly increased capacity to induce mitochondrial depolarisation and oxidative DNA damage compared with micrometric CuO particles. In accordance with the classifications of the International Agency for Research on Cancer (IARC), zinc oxide in non-nanostructured form has been categorised as safe. However, the cytotoxicity and genotoxicity of ZnO nanoparticles have often been associated with their photocatalytic activity (132).

4-2-2- Antimicrobial activity

The antimicrobial properties of MeO-NP are significant, showing notable efficacy against resistant strains and pathogens. microbial resistance, while exhibiting heat resistance that makes them robust antimicrobial agents. (115) In endodontics, the metal oxide nanoparticles most frequently used are characterised by minimal cytotoxicity combined with high biological properties. (98)

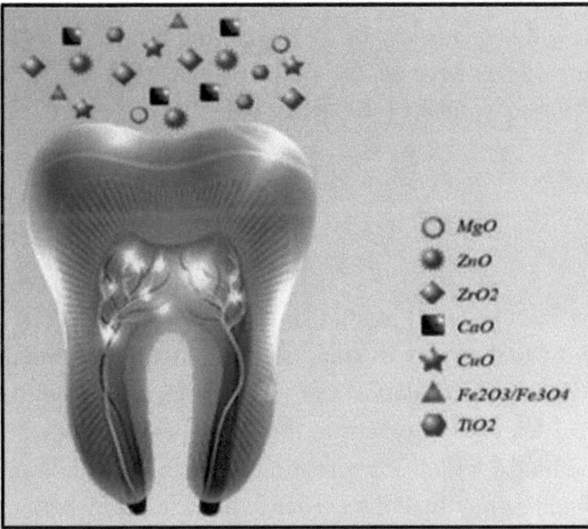

Figure 6: Metal oxide nanoparticles most commonly used in endodontics(98)

Zinc oxide nanoparticles are biocompatible with living organisms and have significant antimicrobial properties. (83) Investigations carried out by Michal Eshed et al. in 2012 (55) examined the behaviour of biofilm on dental surfaces treated with zinc oxide and copper oxide nanoparticles towards Streptococcus mutans. The results revealed a significant reduction in biofilm formation on tooth surfaces coated with ZnO-NP and CuO-NP, with decreases of 85% and 70% respectively, compared with untreated teeth. (98) In their research, Mirhosseini et al. in 2019(96) set out to evaluate the antimicrobial effect of ZnO nanoparticles at different concentrations and sizes against the bacteria E. faecalis, C. albicans, S. mutans and L. fermentum. The observations revealed an increase in the antimicrobial activity of ZnO-NPs as the particle size decreased. In particular, the bacteria C. albicans, E. faecalis and S. mutans showed greater sensitivity to variations in ZnO-NP size than the other microorganisms.

4-2-3- Optical properties

Zinc oxide has interesting characteristics as a transparent material: its refractive index is 2, which contributes to its transparency. It has a strong capacity to absorb and diffuse ultraviolet radiation. When exposed to high-energy sources, such as an intense beam of light or electron bombardment, it emits photons, a process known as luminescence. The luminescence of zinc oxide can be observed in different bands, ranging from the near ultraviolet (around 350 nm) to the visible spectrum, with green emission at a wavelength close to 550 nm (78).

5- Nanoparticles gold

5-1- Definition

Gold nanoparticles (AuNPs) are tiny solids that can be dispersed in a solution, whether aqueous or organic. This dispersion is often referred to as an "inorganic colloidal suspension". (151) However, their electronic configuration is of crucial importance in the context of their clinical applications. Gold is characterised by a high number of electrons per atom (Z = 79). As a result, gold nanoparticles have an exceptional capacity to absorb the energy of X-rays, surpassing that of soft tissue by about 1,000 times (148).

5-2- Properties

5-2-1- Biocompatibility

Semmler-Behnke et al. in 2008,(120) examined the tissue distribution of gold nanoparticles of different sizes in order to analyse the translocation of particles from the respiratory system to the blood after intratracheal instillation and intravenous injections. After 24 hours, 99.8% of the 18 nm AuNP particles were present in the lungs, while 91.5% of the 1.4 nm particles were also found in the lungs, with 8.5% transiting to the liver and bloodstream as secondary targets. (130) These findings highlight the existence of a channel whose access depends on the size of the AuNPs across the air-blood barrier (24).

5-2-2- Antimicrobial activity

Because of their remarkable characteristics, gold nanoparticles are widely recognised as promising antibacterial agents. Their non-toxicity, combined with their functional versatility, makes them particularly attractive for medical applications. What's more, their ability to be functionalised offers the possibility of chemical modifications specifically targeting bacteria. (50)

Compared with AgNPs, gold nanoparticles have weaker antibacterial activity. At high concentrations, AuNPs interact directly with bacterial cells, leading to membrane penetration and ultimately cell lysis. In addition, increasing the surface/volume ratio offers the possibility of improving the antibacterial activity of AuNPs. (24) In endodontics, the current body of studies is insufficient to fully support the efficacy of gold nanoparticles in treatment. Nevertheless, investigations carried out by Bagga et al. in 2017(20) revealed that AuNPs conjugated with levofloxacin were more effective than levofloxacin alone, improving antibacterial activity against Staphylococcus aureus (S.aureus), Escherichia coli and P.aeruginosa(32). A study by Hong et al. in 2015,(85) demonstrated the efficacy of vancomycin-coated nanoparticles against various methicillin-resistant bacterial strains (such as E. faecalis, Enterococcus faecium and S.aureus). Indeed, they were able to inhibit the growth of these strains, underlining their potential as antibacterial agents. (32)

As far as antifungal activity is concerned, it depends mainly on the shape and size of the gold nanoparticles. (24) AuNPs act on both the membrane and cytoplasm of Candida cells. They inhibit the proton pumping necessary for Candida growth and can alter the normal conformation of the cell, resulting in a loss of activity. Small gold nanoparticles with a high surface/radius ratio show increased absorption and better antifungal activity (32).

AuNPs show promising results against pathogens frequently associated with oral diseases and intra-root infections. However, despite these encouraging observations, the studies currently available are not sufficient to fully establish their efficacy compared with silver nanoparticles in terms of antimicrobial effect (32).

6- Nanoparticles from bioverres

6-1- Definition

Bioactive glass (BAG) is an amorphous, highly biocompatible inorganic compound. It is composed of silicon dioxide (SiO_2), sodium oxide (Na_2 O), calcium (CaO) and phosphorus pentoxide (P O_{25}) in various concentrations. (81)

Consequently, bioactive glass nanoparticles (BAG-NP) are small nanometric particles of glass, ranging in size from 20 to 60nm. These nanoparticles have the properties of a bioactive material. This material is one of the most widely used bioactive inorganic materials due to its exceptional biocompatibility and bioactivity. (126)

6-2- Properties

6-2-1- Biocompatibility

In order to assess the biocompatibility of a material, a cytotoxicity test in accordance with ISO10993-5 can be used. (152) The results showed no toxic effect of these materials on the cells. However, it should be noted that bioverres showed a more positive interaction with the cells than the other materials tested. Thus, bioverres powder proved to be biocompatible with cells.

6-2-2- Antimicrobial activity

Nano-sized bioactive glasses have a greater antibacterial effect than ordinary bioactive glass, with the same solid/liquid ratio. In fact, this difference in efficacy is due to the ability of nanoparticles to release almost 10 times more silica into the body fluid than ordinary bioactive glass. conventional glass. In addition, the release of silica has been associated with the antibacterial effect of bioactive glass, and the silica itself also acts as a nucleation site for the immediate precipitation of calcium and phosphate ions (53). Various strategies have been investigated to potentiate the antibacterial properties of BAGs, including the use of specifically formulated antibacterial bioactive glasses, the incorporation of antimicrobial elements such as silver during glass manufacture, and the synergistic combination of bioactive glass with antibiotic agents. (146) (Fig.7)

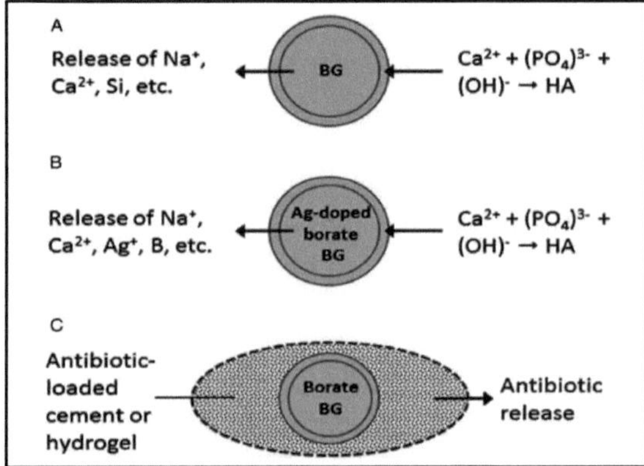

Figure 7: (A) One approach has focused on specially formulated BAGs that can radically alter local physiological conditions when implanted to produce a bactericidal effect.(B) Another approach is to endow the BAG, during manufacture, with minute quantities of elements (e.g. Ag) that are known to have antibacterial activity and, as the glass degrades, these elements are released at a clinically desirable rate.(C) The third approach is to use BAGs in conjunction with antibiotics.(122)

6-2-3- Other properties

In dentistry, bioactive glass nanoparticles are frequently used in regeneration processes because of their affinity for bone tissue, demonstrating exceptional tissue regeneration capacities. Their very structure encourages the formation of new bone tissue (146).

BAG-NP are used effectively in the remineralisation of dentine. When bioactive glass comes into contact with human plasma or saline solution, mineral precipitation by solubility occurs. As a result, an apatite hydroxyl carbonate (HCA) crystallises at the interface between the glass and the tissue, enabling the bone tissue regeneration process to take place due to the similarity between the chemical composition of bioactive glass, human bone and dentin (146).

The introduction of BAG-NP into rat dental pulp stem cells resulted in an increase in the expression of genes associated with odontogenesis and mineralisation capacity. (44) Furthermore, the incorporation of these bioactive nanoparticles into a polymer matrix considerably improves the intrinsically weak mechanical properties of the latter, while preserving its characteristics, such as flexibility, and providing good bioactivity and osteoinductive capacity. (134)

7- hydroxyapatite nanoparticles

7-1- Definition

Hydroxyapatite (Ca_{10} $(PO4)_6$ $(OH)_2$) is a phosphocalcic ceramic with a calcium/phosphorus ratio of 1:67. It is the main component of mineralised tissue, with a significant abundance of calcium phosphates and salts. It predominates in the mineralised tissues of the human body, such as bone and dental enamel, representing around 60-70% and 90% of their weight respectively. (112)
The growing popularity of nanotechnologies in the biomedical field is opening the door to many promising prospects for their practical application in dentistry.

7-2- Properties

Hydroxyapatite (HA) is a calcium phosphate with a chemical structure similar to that of bone mineral, giving it excellent compatibility with biological tissue and high bioactivity. (129)

Biocompatibility is determined by the appropriate response of the host organism, while biological activity refers to the ability of the material to bind to living tissue. (35)

At the nanometric scale, hydroxyapatite nanoparticles (HA-NP) have improved physico-chemical properties compared with conventional hydroxyapatite (35). These nanoparticles have unique properties such as increased solubility, higher surface energy and optimal biological compatibility. (53)

HA-NPs have numerous applications in the biomedical field, notably in regenerative medicine, tissue engineering, dentistry and controlled drug release. Their ability to bind to bone tissue, stimulate cell growth and promote tissue regeneration makes them extremely valuable materials in these fields (92).When considering the therapeutic application of HA-NPs, it is imperative to take into account the biodegradation of these nanometric particles, as

this has a significant influence on the stability of the nanoparticles and the associated physiological response. (92)
A study conducted by Albrecht et al. in 2009 (11) aimed to assess the cytotoxicity of nanometric hydroxyapatite plates of different sizes (45 nm, 90 nm and 100 nm) on primary alveolar macrophages (PAM) and NR8383 cells in rats. The results indicated that the cell viability of PAMs and NR8383 cells was maintained at around 100%. In summary, hydroxyapatite establishes a chemical bond with bone and does not cause any toxicity or inflammation. (92)The nano-hydroxyapatite particles are characterised by a higher remineralising power than a control solution with an equivalent concentration of free ions, demonstrating their ability to promote effective remineralisation. (53)

Because of their biological and chemical similarity to dental structures, HA-NPs can be used to induce dental remineralisation. (53)

These nanoparticles show a significant affinity for association with proteins, plaque fragments and bacteria, due to their small size, which increases the surface area available for protein interactions. In addition, they can function as filling agents, allowing the repair of small cavities and depressions on the surface of tooth enamel. (112)

Bioactivity is another key property of HA-NP. It is considerably high due to its similarity to bone apatite and its high affinity for ion exchange. On the other hand, their biological properties are influenced by the size and morphology of the particles, the type of ionic impurities present in the crystal lattice and the calcium/phosphate (Ca/P) molar ratio, leading to crystallisation in a hexagonal system. (146)
It should be noted that hydroxyapatite nanoparticles can exhibit antimicrobial properties. For example, hydroxyapatite nanosticks loaded with zinc particles release Zn ions^{2+} when used, demonstrating significant antimicrobial activity against oral bacteria. (34) Only at high concentrations can hydroxyapatite nanoparticles exhibit antimicrobial activity in dental materials. (145) However, hydroxyapatite has poor or even mediocre mechanical properties. So, to improve their characteristics, HA-NPs can be doped with elements such as metal ions, which has been shown to reduce the rate of biodegradation. (146)

8- The zirconia

8-1- Definition

Zirconia (Zr), also known as zirconium dioxide, is a white crystalline oxide derived from zirconium. Its crystalline composition is generally 96-99%, excluding any vitreous phase (26) (Fig.8)

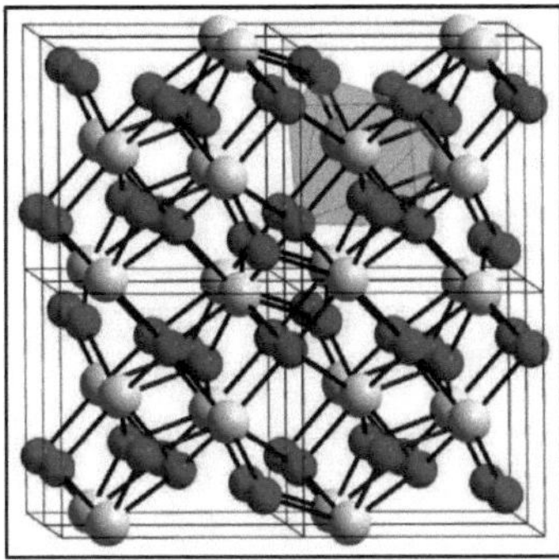

Figure 8: The crystalline structure of zirconium dioxide(153)

This substance is a stabilised regular variant of zirconium oxide. (146) In dentistry, the most commonly used zirconia is stabilised zirconia, also known as yttrium-stabilised tetragonal zirconia (Y-TZP). This material has exceptional mechanical properties and remarkable tear resistance. (26)

8-2- Properties

Various investigations have confirmed that zirconia nanoparticles (Zr- NP) exhibit a toxicity that depends on their concentration. This cytotoxicity results from the oxidative stress generated by ROS. An inhibition of osteoinductive properties was observed by MingfuYe et al. in 2018,(142) at a concentration of 100 mg/ml Zr-NP. Further analysis by Al Zahrani et al. in 2019 (14) also highlighted the deleterious effects of Zr-NP on the DNA of human dermal epithelial cells(26).However, most long-term studies aimed at assessing the cytotoxicity of Zr nanoparticles are limited and lack randomisation. Overall, it should be noted that Zr-NPs have less pronounced toxic effects than titanium oxide and alumina (26).Zirconia-based ceramics, in particular TZP (Tetragonal Zirconia Polycrystals), have excellent mechanical properties. Their flexural strength ranges from 900 to 1200 MPa and their fracture toughness from 7 to 10 MPa m1/2 (26).Zirconia nanoparticles play a significant role in modifying surface energy, as their increased surface area provides more sites for surface-associated activities (26). With this in mind, studies carried out by Mujeeb Khan et al. in 2020, (79) have established that modification of the surface properties of Zr-NP can generate antibacterial activity directed against biofilms. More specifically, the modification of their surface by the addition of glutamic acid, comprising COO^- and NH^+ ions, facilitates the interaction of the ligand with Zr-NP surfaces, thereby enhancing their antibacterial activity. (26) Furthermore, research by Gad et al. in 2017, (58) highlighted a notable antifungal activity of zirconia nanoparticles against the growth of Aspergillus Niger and C.albicans. This ability is attributed to their interference in cell function and the deformation of fungal hyphae. (84) Incorporating Zr-NP into dental materials improves their mechanical properties, such as flexural strength, fracture resistance and hardness, while ensuring satisfactory aesthetics and excellent biocompatibility. Zirconia, with its natural white colour, stable chemical properties, superior corrosion resistance and compatibility with implant materials, is proving to be an effective and efficient ceramic material in dentistry (84).

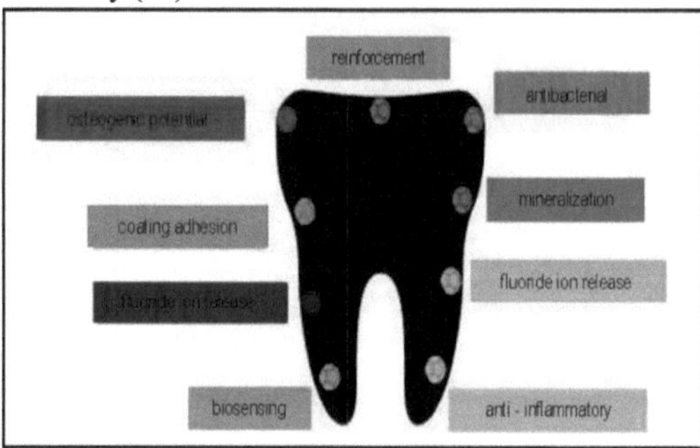

Figure 9: The most significant properties observed following the use of nanomaterials in endodontics(34)

Table I: Summary of the properties of the nanoparticles most commonly used in endodontics.

Properties NPs	Biocompatibility	Antimicrobial	Biological (Healing, Remineralisation...), anti-inflammatory)	mechanical	Other			
					Optics	thermal	electric	Chemical
CS-NP	+	+	+					
G-NP	+	+				+	+	
AgNP	+	++	+		+		+	
MeO-NP (ZnO-NP)	+	+			+			
Au-NP	+-	+						
BAG-NP	++	+-	++					
HA-NP	++	+-	++					
Zr-NP	+-	+-		++				+

Based on the number of research papers published :

Based on the number of scientific papers published :

(++): Nanoparticles (NP) are widely recognised for these properties. (+): Nanoparticles can have these properties.

(+-): Further research is needed to confirm these properties.

CLINICAL APPLICATIONS OF NANOPARTICLES IN ENDODONTICS

1- Preserving pulp vitality

With the aim of preserving the vitality of the dental pulp and encouraging the biosynthetic activity of odontoblastic cells, a conservative approach was adopted.

Pulp capping is a dental procedure designed to protect the pulp in the event of exposure (resulting from deep caries, dental fractures or other injuries) while avoiding more invasive procedures such as endodontic treatment or tooth extraction. To enhance the required properties of the biomaterials used, such as stimulating dentin formation (reactive or reparative), providing an effective seal and promoting pulp healing, nanoparticle technology was applied.

The study by Saghiri et al. in 2018, (119) evaluated the angiogenic properties of some pulp capping materials, such as white MTA (WMTA), calcium hydroxide, Geristore (a resin-modified glass ionomer with a resin-based fluoro alumina silica glass composition) and nano-WMTA. It was noted that the increase in specific surface area with nano-WMTA led to a reduction in setting time and an increase in microhardness. In addition, Geristore and nano-WMTA showed more significant proangiogenic activities. (107)

Akbari et al. in 2013, (10) examined the alterations in the physical properties of the material and the setting time when introducing nano- SiO2 into white mineral trioxide aggregate (WMTA). They found that nano-SiO2, acting as a filler in the cement, improved the microstructure and accelerated the hydration process. (107)

In research led by Li et al. in 2021, (87) Zn-doped Ca-Zn-Si-based bioactive micro-nano glasses were proposed as a material for pulp capping. These materials have demonstrated biocompatible, stimulating odontogenesis and exhibiting significant antibacterial effects. In addition, they activated macrophages to reduce pro-inflammatory markers and promoted dentin remineralisation by stimulating pulp cells. (127) Wang et al in 2021, (138) developed a mineralised film using stable amorphous calcium phosphate nanoparticles (PAsp-ACP), hydroxypropylmethylcellulose (HPMC) and polyaspartic acid. The hydroxyl and methoxy groups present in HPMC were identified as essential contributors to the stability of PAsp-ACP nanoparticles, thus preserving their biomimetic mineralisation capacity. Furthermore, the mineralised membrane demonstrated a propensity to promote early mineralisation of demineralised dentin after 24 hours, with a significant increase in complete mineralisation of demineralised dentin (3-4 µm) observed between 72 and 96 hours. (150)
PLGA-lovastatin nanoparticles, at a concentration of 100 µg/ml, enhance odontoblastic and osteoblastic differentiation, leading to the formation of tubular reparative dentin. However, the effect of PLGA-lovastatin nanoparticles on pulp cells is dose-dependent, highlighting the need for careful evaluation prior to clinical application to determine the appropriate concentration range for direct pulp capping (89). Polymeric hydrogels, mainly composed of carboxymethyl chitosan, were enhanced with calcium phosphate nanoparticles. The resulting product demonstrated an ability to promote the growth of dental pulp stem cells for more than three weeks, with significant osteogenic potential. (106)The superior physical properties of lithium phosphate nanoparticles (Li-MNPs) (their large surface area, larger pore volume, and

a reduced particle size) contributed to enhancing the biomineralisation and odontogenic differentiation of human dental pulp stem cells. Li-MNPs also showed a significant antibacterial effect against S. mutans. These promising results indicate that Li- MNPs have the potential to be used as pulp capping agents. (88)

Recently, BAG-NPs have been loaded with tideglusib (tideglusib/BAG-NP), a thiadiazolidinone known for its inhibitory properties on neurodegeneration and inflammation. This combination aims to optimise the sustained release of tideglusib, thereby improving the bioactivity of the material used for direct pulp capping. (116) Finally, further research and pre-clinical and clinical studies are needed to guarantee the long-term safety and efficacy of these materials.

2- Endodontic irrigation

Endodontic treatment aims to prevent or eliminate microbial invasion of the endo-canal system. It involves a series of steps, including root canal shaping using mechanical instrumentation, abundant endodontic irrigation, followed by a three-dimensional watertight obturation, sealing all communication channels between the root canal system and the periodontium.Effective eradication of the microbial biofilm often plays a decisive role in the outcome of endodontic treatment. However, mechanical treatment alone does not guarantee total disinfection of the root canal. Various irrigation agents such as sodium hypochlorite (NaOCl), ethylenediaminetetraacetic acid (EDTA) and chlorhexidine (CHX) can be used in synergy with instrumentation procedures. (76)

Sodium hypochlorite is commonly used as an endodontic irrigant, frequently at concentrations of between 0.5% and 5.25%. It is considered the gold standard for chemical disinfection of root canals due to its ideal properties. This irrigant is renowned for its antimicrobial potential and its unique ability to dissolve organic tissue. (12, 76)

However, the use of NaOCl can lead to a number of undesirable consequences, including disintegration and weakening of the organic matrix of dentin, reduction in the modulus of elasticity and flexural strength of dentin, causing toxic damage to periapical tissues, and the formation of persistent bacteria. (143)

EDTA is a chelating agent often used to remove dentine sludge. However, excessive use can lead to demineralisation and erosion of dentine, particularly when combined with NaOCl (71).

Chlorhexidine has been suggested as a less caustic endodontic disinfectant and is generally used at a concentration of 2%. It has an antimicrobial effect on a broad spectrum of endodontic flora, and extensive substantivity. (68)

Its main drawbacks are its inability to degrade necrotic tissue and its reduced effectiveness against Gram-negative microbes. (139)

Due to the inherent limitations of conventional endodontic irrigation solutions, more advanced disinfection strategies are being developed and evaluated. The use of NPs is attracting the interest of researchers in the creation of new irrigation materials, with a particular focus on AgNPs, the most widely studied. (117)

- **Silver nanoparticles :**

With regard to endodontic infections, several studies have validated the antimicrobial efficacy of silver nanoparticles against E. faecalis, although their efficacy may be slightly lower than that of sodium hypochlorite. (146) Yin et al. in 2020, (143) suggested that AgNPs at reduced concentration have a biocompatibility superior to that of NaOCl. As an irrigation agent, AgNPs demonstrated comparable efficacy to 2.5% NaOCl and 2% CHX against E. faecalis, suggesting their potential use as a novel intra-channel irrigant. (4)

Another study by Rodriguez et al. in 2018, (118) showed that an AgNP solution destroyed fewer bacteria than a CHX solution, but dissolved more biofilm.(105)

The concept of a multi-purpose solution was tested by Ertem et al. in 2017(54), by developing a solution of porous SiO-coated $AgNPs_2$ in combination with several irrigation solutions, with the aim of preventing biofilm regrowth in endodontic infections.
Unlike conventional treatment approaches involving the sequential use of NaOCl over a wide range of concentrations and EDTA, the all-in-one irrigation solution obtained by simply mixing the two irrigants (NaOCl and AgNP) with chelating agents (such as sodium phytate) offers a one-step alternative, saving significant time. Even after prolonged contact, this new solution showed lower cytotoxicity than the widely used irrigants(4).
Silver nanoparticles can be integrated into the molecular matrix of mesoporous calcium silicate nanoparticles (MCSNN). MCSN-Ag has promising potential as a new intracanal disinfectant due to its significant antibacterial effects and low cytotoxicity(4).

In a study conducted by Ioannidis et al. in 2019,(72) the antimicrobial efficacy of AgNPs synthesised on an aqueous graphene oxide matrix was evaluated. The findings revealed that 2.5 % NaOCl induced maximum biofilm disruption on dentinal tubules, while Ag-GO led to substantial reductions in biovolumes compared to the other experimental groups. In addition, this combination increased stability, prevented aggregation and promoted synergistic antimicrobial properties(4).

The use of ultrasonic activation of Ag-GO also improved antimicrobial action and biofilm disruption in the side channels. (139)

On the other hand, NaOCl can induce toxic damage to periapical tissues, leading to a reduction in the elastic modulus and flexural strength of dentin. In contrast, the use of solutions containing silver nanoparticles had no significant effect on the mechanical properties of dentin. In addition, several studies have confirmed that the application of AgNPs as the final irrigation in root canal therapy increases the fracture resistance of endodontically treated roots(4).The use of an AgNP irrigant containing imidazolium has been associated with an increase in dentin roughness, which may have implications for the adhesion of filling and restorative materials to the root canal walls. (139) The application of the green synthesis method in the production of metallic nanoparticles improves both their biocompatibility and their antimicrobial activity. This improvement was corroborated by the study conducted by Halkai et al. in 2018, (69) which demonstrated that biosynthesised silver nanoparticles exhibited antibacterial activity comparable to that of ampicillin and 2% chlorhexidine against E. faecalis.(139) Diode laser activation of AgNPs represents an innovative method of disinfection applied in endodontics. This approach improves the antibacterial efficacy of

AgNPs without compromising the integrity of tooth structure or periodontal tissues, as demonstrated by the study conducted by Ambalavanan et al. in 2020. (4, 15)

Abbaszadegan et al. in 2015, (2) tested various formulations of silver nanoparticles with different surface charges to compare their antibacterial potential to that of chlorhexidine and sodium hypochlorite. Of all the agents examined, the positively charged silver nanoparticles showed the lowest inhibitory concentration against E. faecalis. These findings highlight the significant impact of surface charge on the antibacterial activity of silver nanoparticles (25).

In summary, antibacterial cationic nanoparticles, in particular AgNPs, show substantial antibacterial activity against biofilms (12).

The efficacy of AgNPs, 2% chlorhexidine, and their combination was evaluated against endodontic pathogens such as E. Faecalis, Klebsiella pneumoniae and C. albicans. The results, from research by Charannya et al. in 2018, (39) revealed that the AgNP-CHX solution exhibits a synergistic effect, resulting in a significant reduction in Escherichia coli colony numbers when applied at a concentration of 70 μg/mL.(4) Another analysis of the antimicrobial efficacy of silver nanoparticles was carried out by Andrade et al. in 2018 (95), showing that the modification of 17% EDTA with AgNPs (EDTA-AgNPs) exerts chelating and antimicrobial effects against C. albicans and S. aureus, both in planktonic cultures and biofilms.(4)

In addition to their direct antibacterial and antifungal efficacy, silver nanoparticles can also potentiate the antibacterial effects of antibiotics against various bacterial strains, including those resistant to antibiotics. This synergistic and multimodal action significantly reduces the need to use high doses of antibiotics, thereby limiting the risk of developing resistance and toxicity for the immune system. (139)

However, it should be mentioned that some bacteria, such as Gram-negative Escherichia coli and Pseudomonas aeruginosa, can rapidly develop resistance to AgNPs after repeated exposure by producing flagellin, which leads to nanoparticle aggregation (139).

AgNPs can also be cytotoxic and tend to aggregate. Their cytotoxicity may be due to the production of ROS, which trigger pro-inflammatory responses in the body. The extent of these responses depends on the concentration, size and aggregation of the AgNPs. However, the use of stabilising agents such as imidazole can prevent AgNP aggregation and mitigate their cytotoxicity, which was confirmed by Abbaszadegan et al. 2015.(2, 139)

Poly (vinyl alcohol) (PVA) was used as a stabilising agent for AgNPs, and this combination showed promising biocompatibility and no genotoxic effect on fibroblast cells. The study by Andrade et al. in 2019, (40) proved the antimicrobial efficacy of PVA-coated silver nanoparticles (AgNP-PVA) in combination with farnesol against various microorganisms, including Enterococcus faecalis, Candida albicans and Pseudomonas aeruginosa. It has been suggested that the use of these AgNP-PVAs in combination with farnesol, after biomechanical preparation, could be considered for root canal disinfection and inhibition of biofilm formation (4, 124).

Nevertheless, some studies have reported the preeminence of conventional endodontic irrigants over silver nanoparticle irrigants. As an example, in vitro investigations conducted by Chang et al. in 2018, (118) revealed that AgNPs used as an irrigant were not found to be effective in removing Enterococcusfaecalis, whereas 2.5% NaOCl was considered a suitable irrigant.Wu et al. in 2014, (140) put forward the idea that the use of silver nanoparticles might be better suited as an intracanal drug due to their interaction and time dependency. They pointed out that the antimicrobial efficacy of AgNPs varied depending on the application technique used.

Treatment with 0.02% AgNP medicated gel was significantly more effective in disrupting biofilm structure than treatment with 0.01% AgNP gel, 0.01% AgNP irrigation solution and calcium hydroxide. These results highlight the importance of selecting the appropriate application method in order to optimise the efficacy of AgNPs in biofilm removal and endodontic infection control. (105, 139)AgNPs are used in endodontics for their unique properties. However, concerns have been raised about their impact on dental aesthetics, due to their potential to stain dentinal walls and cause discolouration,(139) particularly when coated with imidazolium, as confirmed by the study conducted by Moazami et al. in 2018.(97)

Consequently, their use as intracanal irrigants may be restricted due to this adverse effect. However, in the case of posterior teeth, where dental aesthetics are less of a concern, this may not be a problem(4).

In summary, despite the significant antibacterial activity of silver nanoparticles, their use as an intracanal irrigant must be carefully considered because of the prolonged interaction time required to achieve maximum efficacy, as well as the potential toxicity associated with silver ions. A non-toxic concentration must be carefully selected for in vivo application (122).

- **Chitosan nanoparticles :**

Chitosan nanoparticles can be used to improve root canal disinfection in inaccessible root zones and dentinal tubules. (122) However, the use of antibacterial agents within the root canal space faces another challenge: the neutralising effect of different tissue inhibitors. For example, the presence of tissues such as dental pulp and serum albumin significantly inhibited the antibacterial effect of CS-NP. In contrast, dentin, dentin matrix and lipopolysaccharides did not affect the efficacy of these nanoparticles (122). Due to their polycationic nature, CS-NPs exhibit considerable antibacterial efficacy, with increased reactivity at the nanometric scale (135).
It should also be noted that some researchers express uncertainty as to whether the inhibition of bacterial adhesion by chitosan nanoparticles results from the destruction of the surrounding bacteria or from the direct effect of the nanoparticles on the bacterium-substrate interaction. (135)

Studies have shown that irrigating root canals with a solution containing CS-NP for 3 minutes effectively eliminates the dentin sludge present in the root canals. (49) However, final irrigation with CS-NP for 3 minutes led to an alteration in the mineral content of dentine (49).

It is worth pointing out that the chelating effect of both chitosan nanoparticles and EDTA can lead to demineralisation of dentine.
(117) These findings have been corroborated by previous research. They have shown that chitosan-coated dentine surfaces have the potential to remineralise demineralised dentine. (49) Consequently, the use of these nanoparticles has been suggested for the final rinse in root canal irrigation. (117)

The resistance of endodontic infections can be associated with the presence of fungal species. Among these species, Candida albicans is considered to b e one of the most resistant fungi due to its ability to colonise the dentinal walls, penetrate the dentinal tubules and form biofilms (22).

In this study, Balsaraf et al. in 2023, (22) examined the antifungal activity of CS-NPs against Candida albicans. The results revealed that chitosan nanoparticles and 2% CHX solution showed comparable efficacy against C. albicans, while 3% NaOCl solution was significantly more effective than CS-NPs and chlorhexidine. Thus, chitosan nanoparticles could be considered as a potential alternative for endodontic irrigation, offering a solution to the limitations associated with the concentration and time dependency of conventional irrigation solutions such as NaOCl and chlorhexidine on dentin (22).

- **Other nanoparticles :**

Optical coherence tomography (OCT) revealed that incorporating AuNPs and AgNPs into the irrigants used for the root canal improved their biological properties.
The addition of AuNPs is known to reduce micro-infiltration along the canal walls, which improves the adhesion of obturation materials to dentin. Both types of nanoparticles have demonstrated antimicrobial efficacy, reinforcing the ability of the irrigation protocol to reduce the number of bacteria present in the root canal lumen. (131)
Ultrasonic activation is another interesting innovation in endodontics.
Huang et al. in 2023, (71) demonstrated that the use of sonic and ultrasonic agitation of nano-diamond and submicron diamond solutions facilitated the removal of dentinal sludge. In addition, the diamond solution was more effective in the apical region compared with EDTA irrigation.

Combined use of AgNPs and ZnO-NPs in a polymer solution showed superior antimicrobial activity against E. faecalis compared to their use individually, although 2.5% NaOCl was even more effective in reducing bacterial numbers. (139) However, a study by Almeida et al. in 2018, (48) reported slightly lower antimicrobial efficacy of a ZnO- NP based irrigant compared to 2% chlorhexidine and 5% NaOCl.(139) In addition, a study was conducted, by Parolia et al. 2021, (110) to investigate the antibacterial activity of propolis nanoparticles, with an average size of 117.6 nm, as a n irrigant of the root canal infected with E. Faecalis biofilm at a concentration of 300 μg/mL. The results showed that propolis nanoparticles were as effective as 6% NaOCl and 2% chlorhexidine in reducing E. Faecalis biofilm(6).

Nanoparticles of magnesium oxide, titanium dioxide and iron oxide also have antimicrobial properties, although there is less research into their use as potential endodontic irrigants (139).

A study by Jowkar et al. in 2020, (73) demonstrated that final irrigation of canals with nanoparticles of silver, zinc oxide and titanium dioxide improved the fracture resistance (FR) of endodontically treated roots. In an attempt to improve the antiseptic efficacy of conventional endodontic irrigants, a study by Hajihassani et al. 2022, (68) used Nano-CHX gel at a concentration of 2% to overcome the limitations of traditional irrigants used to remove microbial biofilm in the root canal system. The results confirmed that the use of Nano-CHX for endodontic disinfection was as effective as the use of conventional irrigation agents such as 2% chlorhexidine and 5.25% NaOCl. Therefore, Nano-CHX gel can be considered as a promising alternative as a final irrigant, offering high antimicrobial efficacy without the undesirable side effects associated with conventional agents. (68)

3- Instrumentation endodontics

Endodontic rotary instruments, such as nickel-titanium alloy (Ni-Ti) files, are frequently used in dentistry. Nitinol, a Ni-Ti alloy, has an interesting structural feature. It has two distinct crystalline phases, known a s martensite and austenite, and sometimes an intermediate phase known as the R phase. This transition between the martensitic and austenitic phases allows the instruments to retain their elasticity and shape memory, which is essential for optimum performance during endodontic procedures. (146)

It should be noted that nickel-titanium files can be prone to catastrophic failure. Even when subjected to cyclic loads below the yield point, irreversible long-term changes, such as the formation of precipitates and defects, can occur in nickel-titanium alloys (fatigue phenomena), eventually leading to instrument failure.(3)

To minimise the risk of catastrophic failure, nickel-titanium files must be used in accordance with the manufacturer's recommendations, respecting cyclic load limits and avoiding excessive stresses and sudden movements that could compromise their structural integrity.

Nano-indentation is a technique for assessing the performance of Ni-Ti and stainless steel devices.Jamleh et al. in 2011, (73) conducted a study to evaluate the effect of cyclic fatigue on nickel-titanium endodontic instruments using nano-indentation analysis. In this study, a set of Ni-Ti rotary instruments, comprising both new and was subjected to an in-depth analysis. The results showed that nano-indentation is a reliable technique for determining the performance and failure mechanism of instruments. (107)

Adini et al. in 2011 tested the effects of cobalt coatings impregnated with fullerene-type tungsten disulphide (WS2) nanoparticles on the fatigue strength and failure of files(3). All the techniques used - dynamic X-ray diffraction, nano-indentation and torque measurements - demonstrated a significant improvement in the fatigue strength and breakage time of coated endodontic files(3).Coated (fullerene-IF/cobalt-Co) IF/Co files showed reduced friction, phase transformation and mechanical deterioration compared to uncoated files. These results suggest that coated files may be less susceptible to failure under work-related stresses(3).

Various forms of lubricant and irrigation have been developed to reduce friction between endodontic files and the canal surface, helping to reduce the risk of breakage.

Among these solutions, multiwall hollow nanoparticles with an interlocking closed cage, such as IF-WS2 (tungsten disulphide) and IF-MoS2 (molybdenum disulphide), have demonstrated superior tribological behaviour, especially under high loads. Thanks to their near-spherical shape, elasticity and low surface energy, these nanoparticles are proving to be highly suitable solid lubricants(3).

These nanoparticles are marketed under the brand name "NanoLub" as additives to lubricating fluids. They offer significant lubrication benefits(3). A coating a few microns thick, such as the Co/IF coating, can improve the life of endodontic files and potentially allow them to be used without risk of failure. It is important to note that this coating does not alter the mechanical properties of the underlying NiTi alloy, but rather reduces the stresses exerted on the instrument, thereby improving its service life.(3)

4- Medication intracanal

Intracanal medication is a complementary stage in endodontic treatment during which an antibacterial dressing is placed inside the root canal. The aim is to eliminate residual micro-organisms, reduce inflammation and promote healing. This step is generally carried out between treatment sessions to ensure optimum disinfection of the root canal system.

Calcium hydroxide ($Ca(OH)_2$) is the most widely used intracanal medicament, but its efficacy can be altered by a number of factors, including pH, serum proteins, collagen and dentine. Furthermore, its efficacy against E. faecalis and fungi is limited, its anti-inflammatory effect is not very pronounced, and its analgesic power is mixed.

In this context, an evaluation of the antioxidant and anti-inflammatory properties of biosynthesised AgNPs was carried out by Nasim et al. in 2022. (102) The results indicated that, compared with conventional Ca(OH)-based intracanal drugs₂ , biosynthesised AgNPs demonstrated more pronounced antioxidant and anti-inflammatory effects.

The efficacy of silver nanoparticles as drugs, compared to their use as irrigants, demonstrates a significant improvement in the control of bacterial biofilms. Work carried out by Wu et al. in 2014, (140) showed that the application of a medicated gel gel containing 0.02% AgNPs significantly altered the biofilm structure and reduced the number of Enterococcus faecalis cells after treatment, compared with the use of a 0.01% AgNP and calcium hydroxide gel(105).

However, the incorporation of antimicrobial nanoparticles into the compositions of conventional intracanal drugs is attracting increased interest in the field of endodontics.

The addition of AgNP to calcium hydroxide results in a synergistic antimicrobial effect. Balto et al. in 2020, (23) demonstrated that the combination of AgNP and $Ca(OH)_2$, caused a significant reduction in Enterococcus faecalis in the dentine of the root canal. (122)

In addition, this combination promotes synergistic effects that result in improved antimicrobial properties. The antimicrobial activity of the AgNP/$Ca(OH)_2$ combination was more effective than that of calcium hydroxide alone, calcium hydroxide with or without chlorhexidine, and AgNPs alone. However, it was not significantly different from that of the triple antibiotic paste (metronidazole, ciprofloxacin and minocycline). (139)

In addition to their bactericidal action, these silver nanoparticles have shown significant anti-inflammatory and antioxidant effects in the context of endodontic treatment(4).

It has also been reported, by Tanomaruque et al. 2013, (66) that the combination of $Ca(OH)_2$ and ZnO-NP exhibited greater antimicrobial efficacy than ZnO-NP alone. Another study, by Aguiar et al. 2015(8), showed that the addition of chlorhexidine further enhanced the antimicrobial properties of this $Ca(OH)_2$ /ZnO-NP combination.(139) In the same context, the research results of Shahi et al. in 2018, (144) showed that the application of calcium hydroxide with silver, copper, zinc or magnesium indicated that the combination of 1%

copper and calcium hydroxide paste appeared to be the most effective.(105) Thus, the combination of chlorhexidine with AgNPs has been shown not only to enhance antibacterial activity, but also to amplify the residual antibacterial effect of CHX as an intracanal drug. These synergies have demonstrated a significant residual antibacterial effect against Enterococcus faecalis, making these combinations potential candidates as intracanal drugs for use between treatment sessions, effectively preventing bacterial regrowth.(5)

Calcium nanohydroxides have several advantages over their conventional form. Their smaller size means they are better able to penetrate the dentinal tubules, resulting in more effective antibacterial activity against E. faecalis (139).

In addition, the use of calcium nano-hydroxides results in a lesser reduction in dentin microhardness compared with conventional calcium hydroxide. With regard to fracture resistance, the application of nanocalcium hydroxides causes a lesser reduction compared to conventional calcium hydroxide. (139)

Iffat Nasim et al. in 2022, (101) evaluated the microhardness of root dentin after the use of an intra-canal drug. Different drug combinations were tested, namely a $CaOH_2$ /AgNP combination, an AgNP/GO combination, and a control group using calcium hydroxide alone. The GO/AgNP-based intracanal drug had the least effect on root dentin microhardness compared with the other combinations (101).
Although numerous studies have reported the effectiveness of using silver nanoparticles in endodontic medication, other studies have reported less conclusive results.It is essential to stress that when applying AgNPs, it is imperative to restrict their use to the root canal space and to meticulously ensure that any residue is removed from the pulp chamber before restoring the crown(4).

Nanoparticulate calcium silicate compounds with internal porous structures are attracting increased interest because of their bioactive, biocompatible and osteogenic properties, as well as their substantivity and potential as drug carriers. (139)

Further studies have also shown that mesoporous calcium silicate nanoparticles combined with AgNPs or ZnO-NPs exhibit high antibiofilm efficacy, minimal cytotoxicity, sustained ion release, infiltration into dentinal tubules and negligible changes in the mechanical properties of dentin (139).

Another intracanal drug, chlorhexidine, has been shown to alter dentin structure, leading to a decrease in dentin microhardness. Therefore, the impact of nano-chlorhexidine was investigated in the study conducted by Naseri et al. in 2019. (100) The results confirmed that nano-CHX did not cause any change in microhardness, although a change in chemical structure was observed one week after application of the two substances. (107)

Chitosan nanoparticles, due to their significant antimicrobial properties, have been used in the context of intracanal medication. The incorporation of these nanoparticles into a Ca(OH)-based $paste_2$ offers the potential to improve the capacity for penetration of the paste into the dentinal tubules, resulting in increased antibacterial activity. (124 In addition, CS-NPs were found to be less damaging to dentin strength than calcium hydroxide, due to their ability to promote collagen cross-linking and neutralise matrix metalloproteinases. (139) The properties of bioactive glass nanoparticles as potentially effective agents against biofilm in root canals have been extensively studied. The results of an analysis, conducted by Obeid et al. 2021, (104) revealed that BAG-NP demonstrated the greatest antimicrobial activity, followed by BAG and Ca(OH)2 . However, it is important to note that, despite their potential, none of these drugs succeeded in completely eliminating E. faecalis.

Graphene oxide has demonstrated promising antimicrobial properties against a broad spectrum of micro-organisms, in addition to its ability to transport antibiotics.

A study conducted by Eskandari et al. in 2023, (56) aimed to compare the antibacterial activity of dual antibiotic paste (DAP), graphene oxide alone, as well as their combination (GO-DAP), against Enterococcus faecalis. GO-DAP demonstrated persistent antibacterial efficacy against E. faecalis, making it a promising option as an intracanal drug for root canal treatment.

5- Root canal filling

5-1- Cements for sealing

ZOE cements are mainly composed of zinc oxide and eugenol. It offers a number of advantages, such as biocompatibility, activity antibacterial properties, easy filling of the space between the gutta- percha cone and the walls of the root canal, and a good seal.

However, ZOE luting cement also has some disadvantages, including shrinkage during setting and dissolution in tissue fluids. It can also be relatively slow setting, which may require a prolonged curing time. In addition, it is sensitive to moisture and therefore requires a dry environment during application.

As a result, a new endodontic sealant, called NZOE, has been developed, incorporating nanoscale particles of ZOE powder. This formulation is designed to improve the physicochemical and antimicrobial properties, optimise the performance of the material, and overcome some of the drawbacks associated with traditional ZOE-based sealants. (139)

A comparative study, conducted by Zarei (147) et al. in 2018,revealed the antimicrobial activity of NZOE sealing cement compared to two other commonly used endodontic sealers, namely AH26 (resin-based) and Pulpdent (zinc oxide eugenol-based). The study evaluated their efficacy against endodontic pathogens such as E. faecalis, S. mutans, S. aureus, E. coli and C. albicans at different time intervals.

The results showed that NZOE had the highest antimicrobial activity. It succeeded in eliminating all the micro-organisms tested, with the exception of one strain of E. faecalis colony, which was reduced to zero after treatment.
2 hours. In contrast, the AH26 and Pulpdent sealers failed to completely eliminate the E. faecalis colony throughout the observation period. (147)

Chitosan nanoparticles have been studied in the context of endodontic sealants. The use of CS-NPs to modify sealants at based on zinc oxide and eugenol, has led to an improvement in their antibacterial and anti-biofilm properties (139). Da Silva et al. in 2013, (47) used a zinc oxide and eugenol-based sealant incorporated with CS-NPs for in vitro obturation of root canals in treated cattle. This modification of the sealant inhibited biofilm formation at the sealant-dentin interface.Furthermore, a study byDel carpio et al. in 2015,(37) demonstrated that incorporating CS-NP into an epoxy resin (ThermaSeal, York, PA) enhanced their antimicrobial activity through direct contact and membrane restriction. Furthermore, a reduction in biofilm formation at the sealant-dentin interface was observed, even after a four-week ageing period (122).

The incorporation of CS-NP and ZnO-NP into a resin-based endodontic sealer improved the antibacterial properties of the material and its ability to diffuse antibacterial compounds. The addition of these nanoparticles did not alter the flow characteristics of the sealer in the root canal. (122)

In addition, CS-NP can be combined with calcium phosphate compounds, bringing their chemical composition and crystalline structure closer to the apatitic materials found in teeth and bone. This improves the adhesion of the sealant to dentin. However, there are also limitations to the use of chitosan nanoparticles, particularly during endodontic reprocessing (146).

Comparative analysis by S. Pattanaik et al. in 2019, (111) highlighted that the addition of chitosan to AH Plus sealant exhibited superior antifungal properties compared to Apexit Plus and MTA Fillapex sealants. These results highlight the beneficial potential of chitosan in as an additive in endodontic sealants to combat fungal infections. (146)

Quaternary ammonium compounds, particularly quaternary ammonium polyethyleneimine (QPEI), have been studied as antibacterial agents in dental materials and root canal sealants. QPEI nanoparticles have demonstrated broad antimicrobial and antibiofilm activity by interacting electrostatically with bacterial cell membranes, causing cell damage and the release of cellular constituents. In addition, their insoluble nature gives them long-term antimicrobial efficacy. QPEI, when incorporated into epoxy resin-based sealants, imparts an antimicrobial property to these materials, making them suitable as antibacterial biomaterials. (139) The results of tests carried out by Barros et al. in 2014, (28) demonstrated that incorporating 1% of QPEI nanoparticles into sealants improves the antimicrobial effect of these products, particularly against bacteria present in the oral cavity.(122) Other studies have demonstrated the possibility of combining QPEI nanoparticles with commercial sealants without altering their biocompatibility or physicochemical properties such as solubility, flow, compressive strength and dimensional stability. However, the incorporation of QPEI nanoparticles into AH Plus™ did not result in a significant improvement in its antibacterial efficacy, although strain-dependent antibiofilm effects were observed. In contrast, the addition of QPEI nanoparticles to Pulp Canal Sealer™ improved its antibacterial and antibiofilm efficacy against E. faecalis (122, 146). In addition, Gong et al. in 2014, (63) developed a material designed to prevent reinfections and combat endodontic infections during root filling. They enriched AH Plus with ammonium epoxy silicate (QAES) with a rough surface, a spherical shape and a diameter of around 120 nm. The researchers observed that this material was effective for in vivo disinfection of the root canal after obturation. (146) Dimethylaminohexadecyl methacrylate (DMAHDM) is another chemical variant of quaternary ammonium. Its structure is composed of a long chain that can be in a resin matrix after bond formation by root polymerisation. (139) A study conducted by Seung et al. in 2018, (121) modified the epoxy resin-based AH Plus™ by adding DMAHDM and AgNPs, which led to a significant improvement in antimicrobial properties. Unlike AH Plus™ which lost its antibacterial efficacy after 7 days, the modified sealant maintained its antibacterial properties for 14 days. (139)

In a promising approach by Baras et al. in 2019, (27) an experimental sealant containing amorphous calcium phosphate (nACP) nanoparticles associated with DMAHDM, was evaluated. This sealant demonstrated significant antibiofilm activity and a high release of calcium and phosphate ions, suggesting a potential to promote remineralisation and strengthen weakened root structures.(6)In the study by Chang et al. in 2020,(38) a new root canal sealant was developed using urethane acrylates based on polycarbonate polyol (PCPO), a macrodiol prepared from carbon dioxide. To reinforce the seal's antibacterial effect, wafers of nanometric silicate (NSP) were used, to which silver nanoparticles and/or zinc oxide nanoparticles were immobilised. Antibacterial efficacy was assessed using Enterococcus faecalis as the test microorganism. The results showed that PCPO-based acrylate urethanes containing 50 ppm AgNP and ZnO-NP immobilised on silicate wafers, called Ag/ZnONSP, exhibited good biocompatibility and enhanced antibacterial activity.

Inaam Baghdadi et al. in 2021, (21) modified BioRoot™ RCS, a bioceramic sealer used for root canal sealing, by adding three different types of nanoparticles: multiwall carbon nanotubes (MWCNTs), titanium carbides (TCs) and boron nitrides (BNs). The results obtained indicated that the addition of 1 wt% MWCNT and TC significantly improved the compressive strength and microstructure of the initial BioRoot™ RCS.

5-2- Material filling root canal (Gutta percha)

Although gutta-percha is the most widely used root canal filling material, its antimicrobial properties are limited, which may compromise the elimination of residual bacteria in the canal. In addition, its effect on the fracture resistance of endodontically treated roots is still being debated and questioned.Advances in root canal filling materials aim to fill the gaps associated with gutta-percha by improving antimicrobial properties and fracture resistance. The integration of nano-sized agents offers new prospects for more effective and durable root canal fillings. (139)In the study conducted by Alves et al in 2018, (13) a novel approach was used to improve the antimicrobial efficacy of commercial Gutta-percha (GP) cones. Two methods were explored to enhance the antibacterial properties of GP cones.

In the first stage of this study, the GP was coated with AgNP. The results obtained showed a significant improvement in the antibacterial and antifungal properties of gutta- percha coated with silver nanoparticles. In addition, this modification showed significant efficacy in preventing bacterial leakage. In a second step, the surface of another group of GPs underwent argon plasma treatment, followed by the deposition of a thin layer of ZnO. The results showed that the plasma treatment considerably improved the surface properties of the GP cones, such as the specific surface/volume ratio, free energy and reactivity. The modified GP cones showed superior antibacterial activity compared with untreated GP cones, and this activity was further enhanced by the ZnO deposition. The conventional disinfection protocol using sodium hypochlorite altered the surface of the GP cones, resulting in irregular topography and abundant deposits. In addition, the direct deposition of ZnO on virgin GP cones also produced a rough surface. However, with plasma treatment, the GP cones showed improved surface properties (13).

In a study conducted by Singh et al. in 2021, (123) a new polymer nanocomposite was developed to enhance the mechanical and antimicrobial properties of the material. The researchers coated this polymer with nanoplatelets of reduced graphene oxide (GNP).

The graphene nanoplatelets embedded in the polymer had mechanical properties comparable to those of gutta-percha. gutta-percha, with a tensile strength of 27-36% and an elongation at break of 2.1-3.1%. In addition, GNP demonstrated superior antimicrobial activity, significantly inhibiting bacterial colonisation compared with commercial gutta-percha, while preserving the integrity of surrounding cells. These results highlight the potential advantages of this material in terms of mechanical strength and antimicrobial action for application as an endodontic filling material (123).

Another study, by Lee et al. in 2015, (86) also investigated modifications to gutta-percha by incorporating ND nanodiamonds for filling the middle third of root canals. NDs, with a size of approximately 46 nm, offer unique advantages due to their favourable properties for dental applications, including their versatile surface chemistry, biocompatibility and mechanical properties. In addition, these nanodiamonds are coated with amoxicillin, which can improve the efficacy of endodontic therapies by eliminating microbes and preventing reinfection of the root canal. The incorporation of ND has also enhanced the mechanical strength of the gutta-percha cones, making them easier to handle clinically.

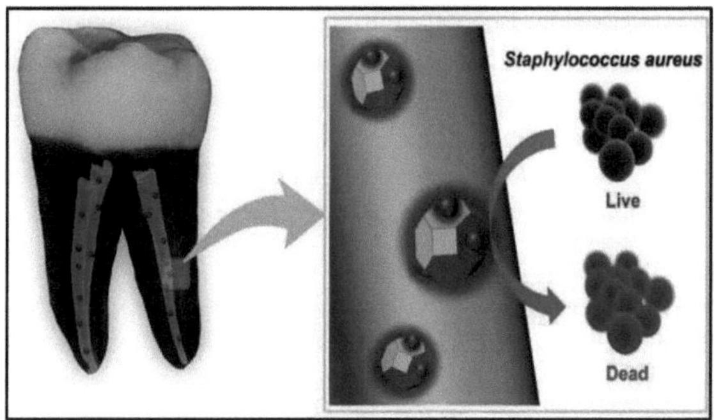

Figure 10: Schematic representation of gutta-percha treated with nanodiamonds and coated with amoxicillin(86).

6- Regeneration pulp

Nanoparticles have attracted increasing interest due to their potential to improve the outcome of the pulp regeneration process. The properties of nanoparticles, such as their ability to release bioactive molecules in a controlled manner, their high bioavailability and their ability to penetrate tissue, make them attractive candidates for pulp regeneration applications.

CS-NPs have been shown to be effective in several studies focusing on dental pulp regeneration. The synergistic use of scaffolds and odontogenic inducing factors creates a favourable environment for dental pulp and dentin regeneration by dental pulp stem cells. (146) Nanoparticles have been adapted to create different forms of scaffolds (temporary structures designed to mimic the extracellular matrix and provide support for stem cell and tissue growth and differentiation), which play an essential role in regenerative endodontic therapies. (70)

In addition, scaffolds can be combined with carrier systems, known as nanocarriers, enabling the controlled release of different bioactive molecules. Nanocarriers can be loaded with specific molecules and released in a programmed manner, improving the efficiency and precision of regenerative treatment. (70)

Elgendy et al. in 2017, (52) investigated natural scaffolds such as propolis and chitosan. They showed the potential of these scaffolds for endodontic treatment due to their biocompatibility and ability to promote tissue regeneration. (125) In a study by Bellamy et al. in 2016, (31) a carboxymethylchitosan-based scaffold loaded with chitosan nanoparticles containing transforming growth factor-β1 was used to improve the viability, differentiation and migration of apical papilla stem cells (APSCs)(139).

In addition, the use of CS-NP loaded with bovine serum albumin improved SCAP viability and increased alkaline phosphatase (ALP) activity. (135)

Similarly, the incorporation of chitosan nanoparticles loaded with dexamethasone produced improvements in the odontogenic differentiation of SCAPs. (139)

In recent research conducted by Bhaskar et al. in 2021, (29) porous nano-HAs derived from eggshell and carboxymethyl cellulose revealed a significant increase in the expression of vascular endothelial growth factor (VEGF) and dentin sialophosphoprotein, highlighting their potential in promoting tooth regeneration.(125)The role of AuNPs in pulp regeneration was evaluated by Biz et al. in 2019. (33) They incorporated AuNPs with a biodegradable organic plastic, L-lysine, to facilitate their internalisation by stem cells.

Furthermore, the incorporation of 0.2 mg/ml AuNP-PLL did not interfere with the baseline behaviour of dental pulp stem cells (DPSC). This methodology therefore proves to be a useful tool for cell labelling to observe cell behaviour and interaction with 3D scaffolds, opening up a range of new approaches in regenerative endodontics. Hydroxyapatite nanoparticles have found wide application in the field of odontogenic regeneration. When in contact with pulp tissue, HA stimulates regeneration by encouraging the formation of complex cells and tissues. What's more, hydroxyapatite integrates harmoniously into the bone without causing toxicity, immune response, infection or inflammation. (18)

Incorporation of HA-NP into the scaffolds promoted the differentiation of DPSCs into the odontoblast-like phenotype, as demonstrated by in vitro and in vivo studies. One study also evaluated the differentiation of human odontogenic DPSCs on poly L-lactic acid (PLLA) fibres and showed promising results. (146) Tondnevis et al. in 2019, (130) explored the fabrication of a dental tissue scaffold by incorporating nano-hydroxyapatite or nano-fluoro-hydroxyapatite (nano-FHA) with chitosan. The results showed that the addition of chitosan to the scaffold led to a significant increase in cell proliferation. (125) In the field of dental pulp regeneration, the plant extract ElaeagnusAngustifolia (EA) was used to modify nano-hydroxyapatite and assess its impact on the differentiation of dental pulp stem cells.Azaeyan et al. in 2023, (19) showed that incorporation of HA-NP modified by EA extract (nHAEA) into a poly(epsilon- caprolactone) (PCL) composite improved cellular and intercellular adhesion. In addition, nHAEA stimulated the expression of human leukocyte antigen-G5 (HLA-G5), vascular endothelial growth factor (VEGF), dentin sialophosphoprotein (DSPP) and interleukin 6 (IL6) genes. These results suggest that nHAEAs could have a potential application in the treatment of dental pulp. by improving the regenerative capacity of DPSCs. (19) These studies open up new prospects for the development of dental regenerative therapies based on the use of nanomaterials and plant extracts. (19) The impact of bioactive nano-glass (58S) on the odontogenic differentiation and mineralisation of human dental pulp cells was examined by Gong et al. in 2014.(64) In their in vitro study, they observed that bioactive nano-glass more effectively promoted the differentiation and mineralisation of human dental pulp cells.(107)

In addition, studies have shown that odontogenic differentiation of human dental pulp cells can be stimulated by incorporating dexamethasone and bioactive glass nanoparticles into a nanofibre scaffold system (139).Another approach was to reinforce the hydrogel scaffolds using cellulose nanocrystals. This method increased the rigidity and stability of the scaffolds. In addition, the reinforced hydrogel was enriched with platelet lysate containing proangiogenic and chemotactic factors, which has the potential to improve pulp tissue revascularisation and regeneration. (139) Exosomes have attracted growing interest due to their high potential for promoting intercellular communication, enhanced cell recruitment, differentiation towards specific cell lineages and tissue repair. Exosomes are small extracellular vesicles (30-90 nm) containing various bioactive molecules such as DNA, RNA, lipids and proteins. MicroRNAs (miRNAs), in particular, have been shown to have a positive effect on exosomes. increasingly recognised for their role in regulating cellular processes and their therapeutic potential. The aim of the study conducted by Ganesh et al. in 2022,(60) was to evaluate the effect of exosomes on cell orientation and angiogenic differentiation for dental pulp regeneration. Exosomes (DPSC-Exos) were isolated from rabbit dental pulp stem cells cultured under conditions of growth (Exo-G) or angiogenic differentiation (Exo-A). DPSC-Exos showed a significant improvement in cell proliferation and migration when treated with a specific concentration of exosomes. In addition, gene expression analysis revealed that DPSC-Exos enhanced the expression of angiogenic markers such as vascular endothelial growth factor A (VEGFA), Fms-related tyrosine kinase 1 (FLT1) and platelet-endothelial cell adhesion molecule 1 (PECAM1). The microRNAs contained in Exo-A exosomes have been identified as playing a key role in cell orientation and angiogenesis. These results suggest that the exosome-based cell orientation and angiogenic differentiation strategy has significant therapeutic potential for dental pulp regeneration. These advances open up promising new prospects for the development of innovative regenerative therapies in endodontics, with the possibility of encouraging the regeneration of dental tissue. These developments offer advanced solutions for patients requiring endodontic treatment.

7- Coronal filling materials [107]

Coronal fillings following endodontic treatment are of crucial importance for the preservation, functional restoration and aesthetic improvement of the treated tooth. Coronal restorative materials must have certain fundamental properties, such as good adhesion to the tooth, low thermal conductivity, dimensional stability, adequate setting time, acceptable aesthetics, satisfactory mechanical strength, and so on. In addition, they are classified into two main categories: direct and indirect restorative materials.However, a major problem with modern coronal restorative materials is the loss of watertightness, which leads to microbial infiltration and recurrent caries, and eventually to the failure of endodontic treatment. The durability of adhesion between resin-based composites and dentine is not optimal, limiting the longevity of adhesive restorations to just a few years.

Thus, the application of nanotechnology in restorative dentistry, combined with the integration of nanoparticles, not only offers the prospect of improving the strength and longevity of restorations, but is also likely to counter the appearance of secondary caries by conferring antibacterial properties on coronal restorations.

7-1- Resins composites

A range of nanoparticles used in the development of nanocomposites have demonstrated their ability to optimise the physical properties of composite resins, while preserving their radiopacity.

Investigations on composite resin discs showed that the introduction of AgNP at a concentration of 0.35% inhibited the growth of S. mutans and Lactobacillus acidophilus without compromising their compressive strength or altering their surface roughness (103). Recently, studies have shown that the incorporation of silver nanoparticles into commercial microhybrid resin composites has resulted in an increase in the contact angle at the surface of the materials, leading to a reduction in the adhesion and proliferation of pathogenic bacteria. However, the synthesis and dispersion of these silver nanoparticles present challenges due to their tendency to agglomerate. (30)

In an attempt to overcome these problems, cross-linked dimethacrylate/silver nanohybrid composites were synthesised by coupling photopolymerisation particles, resulting in 3 nm nanoparticles that were well dispersed in the matrix, without altering the mechanical properties of the material. However, these results are only reliable for very low concentrations (0.02%) of AgNP, while at higher concentrations, these nanoparticles had no beneficial effect on the antibacterial capacity of resin composites and appeared to compromise the photopolymerisation of the restorative material. (30)

In another approach, AgNPs were combined with an antibiotic, Ciprofloxacin (CIP), in order to potentiate the antibacterial action of composite resins. Arif et al. in 2022, (17) showed that resin composites containing CIP-AgNP exhibited increased antibacterial activity and better compressive strength than standard resin composites. In addition, these composites were more biocompatible than those containing only AgNPs and had no negative effect on dental aesthetics.Zinc oxide nanoparticles were incorporated into a composite resin in order to evaluate their efficacy as an antibacterial agent. Wang et al. in 2019, (137) pointed out that, in addition to their anti-adhesive and antibacterial activity against S. mutans, composite resins modified with ZnO-NP have maintained their mechanical properties. This characteristic offers significant advantages not only in the prevention of secondary caries, but also in the fracture resistance of the material (113). A study carried out by Teymoornezhad et al. in 2016, (128) showed that incorporating 3% zinc oxide nanoparticles into a fluid resin composite had the effect of reducing microleakage phenomena. (113)

In a comparison of antibacterial properties between composite resins containing 1% AgNPs and those incorporating 1% ZnO-NPs, it was observed that resins with ZnO-NPs showed significantly greater antibacterial activity against Streptococcus mutans than those containing AgNPs. (124)The incorporation of spherical zirconia nanoparticles showed an effective barrier against crack propagation in the hybrid layer during microtensile strength tests. In addition, improvements in nanohardness and nano-elasticity within the hybrid layer were observed for up to 3 months with the addition of zirconium chloride nanoparticles (30).

In addition, the incorporation of AuNP improved the mechanical properties of the resins without causing toxicity to the cells (24).

However, it should be noted that the incorporation of these nanoparticles can lead to a reduction in light transmission, which can give an opaque appearance to the restoration. This should be taken into account when using them in aesthetic dental applications. (24)

More recently, an innovative magnetic dental composite material has been evaluated, based on the use of coated magnetite nanoparticles. a double layer of silicon dioxide (SiO2) and calcium hydroxide Ca(OH)2 . This material has the ability to induce local calcification and promote the formation of secondary dentine, while also displaying bacteriostatic properties, making it particularly promising for specific applications in dentistry (45).

The use of nanodiamonds functionalised with a quaternised copolymer within resin composites has demonstrated an ability to inhibit biofilm formation without altering the structural integrity of the tooth. This advance could be of significant importance in preventing infections and failures associated with dental restorations. (94)

A study conducted by Chung et al. 2016, (43) successfully created a nanocomposite by mixing HA nanoparticles (inorganic constituent, 75 wt%) with chitosan (organic constituent, 25 wt%). This mixture of components mimics the physiological composition of teeth, which can improve the performance and integration of the composite into the dental structure. (125)

Advances in research have led to the development of innovative strategies for repairing cracks and eradicating dental caries using triple agents. These agents include self-healing microcapsules, dimethylaminohexadecyl dimethacrylate (DMAHDM), and amorphous calcium apatite nanoparticles (nACP). This innovative approach is applicable to a variety of dental materials, including adhesives, cements, sealants and composites. (94) In a study conducted by Cao et al. in 2017, (36) a resin containing silver nanoparticles was developed using AgBr/BHPVP nanocomposites. This resin exhibited a continuous release of Ag+ ions which exerted a particularly potent antibacterial effect on Streptococcus mutans, while preserving the material's flexural strength and modulus (94).A study by Xiao et al. in 2017,(141) led to the design of a bioactive multifunctional composite (BMC) incorporating nanoparticles of nACP, MPC (2-methacryloyloxyethylphosphorylcholine), DMAHDM, and AgNP. The incorporation of poly(amido amine) (PAMAM) into the BMC gave it powerful antibacterial properties(94). This study focused on the remineralisation of root dentin and demonstrated that BMC + PAMAM is effective in protecting tooth root structures and holds promise for restorations of different classes of tooth cavities, including Class I and Class II restorations (94).

These materials could revolutionise dentistry by providing more effective and durable restorative options for preserving oral health. However, further research will be needed to confirm their long-term safety and efficacy before their widespread clinical use.

A number of research studies have looked at incorporating nanometric fillers into dental composites to reinforce their structure and give them antibacterial properties. In a study conducted by Wang et al. 2018, (136) wrinkled mesoporous silica nanoparticles (WMS), was introduced into unimodal and bimodal fillers. The results indicate that WMS associated with a bimodal filler blend exhibits improved mechanical properties compared with its counterpart with a unimodal filler blend. This innovative approach made it possible to increase the composite's strength while preserving its fundamental clinical characteristics. (94) Research conducted by Ai et al. 2017, (9) aimed to reinforce dental composites using hydroxyapatite (HA) nanowires coated with polydopamine (PDA) and treated with silver nanoparticles. The modified HA-PDA-Ag nanowires exhibited remarkable adhesion to the Bis-GMA resin matrix, as well as effective antibacterial activity. The resulting composite exhibited substantial bactericidal activity without causing toxicity to surrounding tissues, qualifying it as a particularly suitable nanofiller for dental applications. (94) Other research has recommended the use of composites containing CaP nanoparticles in areas where total removal of caries tissue is not recommended. In addition, they are indicated for early carious lesions and in patients at high risk of caries, such as those with xerostomia. (30)In terms of clinical performance, studies have reported that nanocomposites have properties and results comparable to, or even better than, those of hybrid and microfilled composites. Nanocomposites have shown promise for occlusal restorations and pit and fissure sealants, demonstrating their effectiveness in caries prevention. (30)

7-2- Glass ionomer cements CVI

Glass ionomer cements (GICs) are materials widely used in dentistry, particularly for their fluoride ion release properties, which help prevent secondary caries. These cements can be modified by incorporating nanoparticles to improve their mechanical and antibacterial properties.With the aim of improving the mechanical properties without compromising the clinical characteristics of CVI, Rehman et al. 2008, (99) demonstrated that the addition of polyacids containing N-vinylpyrrolidone (NVP), as well as nano-HA and fluoroapatite (nano-FA), to conventional glass ionomer (Fuji II, GC International, Tokyo, Japan) improved its mechanical strength compared to commercial Fuji II cement. (133)

The incorporation of titanium dioxide nanoparticles into CVI also improved its mechanical properties and antibacterial activity against Streptococcus mutans (133).

In addition, copper-doped CVI has demonstrated increased antibacterial efficacy and reduced collagen degradation (94).The findings of the study conducted by Paiva et al. 2018, (108) revealed that AgNP-enriched CVI demonstrated exceptional antibacterial activity against Streptococcus mutans. (94)

Resin-modified glass ionomer cements (RIMVC) are used in a variety of clinical applications, including temporary fillings on permanent teeth, liners or bases, sealants, dentine substitutes, particularly for cervical fillings, and root caries. (133)

The integration of nanoparticles into CVIMAR by 3M ESPE has given rise to a new category of restorative materials known as nanoionomers. These nanoionomers include copolymers of acrylic acid and itaconic acid, aluminosilicate glass, bisphenol A-glycidyl methacrylate, triethylene glycol dimethacrylate, hydroxyethyl methacrylate and nanofillers. (133)

7-3- Dental adhesives

To improve the long-term clinical performance of resin composites, efforts have focused on reducing the effects of polymerisation shrinkage and the viscosity of highly filled materials.

Degradation of the hybrid layer in dental adhesives is mainly the result of hydrolytic and enzymatic degradation processes affecting the collagen fibrils and the hydrophilic resin. Various approaches have been used to counteract this degradation, including the incorporation of nanoparticles of amorphous calcium phosphate, bioactive glass or hydroxyapatite into dental adhesives. (30)

The incorporation of AgNPs had no significant impact on adhesives applied to non-carious dentin. However, it did lead to a substantial decrease in biofilm viability and metabolic activity, as well as a reduction in colony-forming units and lactic acid production when AgNPs were introduced into the adhesive (103).

Several studies have shown that the addition of ZnO-NP to dental adhesives considerably improves their quality. The incorporation of these nanoparticles into dental adhesive systems has been associated with a significant improvement in their antimicrobial properties, while preserving their adhesive strength. (113)

Dadkan et al. 2014, (46) investigated the influence of gold nanoparticles on dentin bond strength in an experimental bonding agent. In addition, the addition of graphene nanoplatelets led to an improvement in the flexural and tensile strength of the dental adhesive, with optimum concentrations set at 10X for flexural strength and 5X for tensile strength. (24)

A strong and stable dentin hybrid layer must be able to withstand the cyclic stresses imposed on the restorative interface, while maintaining high initial bond strength values. The incorporation of spherical zirconia nanoparticles has been identified as generating an effective barrier against crack propagation from the base of the hybrid layer in microtensile strength tests. (30)

In addition, the incorporation of HA-NP into bonding agents has been studied to improve the biomechanical properties of the adhesive resin, thereby reinforcing tooth structure and durability (30). The joint use of nano-amorphous calcium phosphate (nACP) with quaternary ammonium dimethacrylate (QADM) and nanosilver (nAg) in dentin adhesives aims to take advantage of the benefits of different approaches. This combination seeks to remineralise demineralised collagen while reducing the presence of bacteria around the adhesive interface (30).

Experimental dentin adhesives containing nanogels based on UDMA or bisphenol-A dimethacrylateethoxylated (BisEMA) (particle size 10-80 nm) have shown that the size of the nanogel particles allows them to be dispersed in the dentin tubules and sometimes in the interfibrillar spaces. The addition of nanogel limits oxygen diffusion rates at the surface of the material, thereby reducing oxygen inhibition during polymerisation of the adhesive layer. However, the level of hydrophilicity of the nanogel impacts not only its mechanical performance but also the strength of adhesion to dentin and the stability of the restorative material over time (30).In summary, the incorporation of nanoparticles into dental adhesives is emerging as a promising strategy for optimising their mechanical, antibacterial and remineralising characteristics. However, careful consideration of nanoparticle dispersion is crucial to ensure their effectiveness in the context of dental restorations.

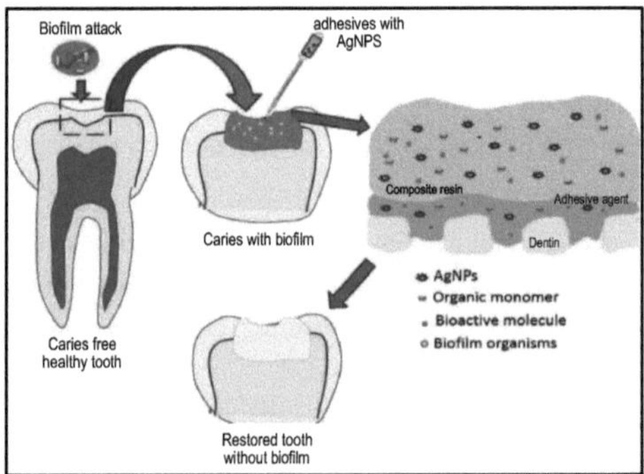

Figure 11: Incorporating AgNPs into composite resins and adhesive systems eradicates biofilm organisms, prevents microleakage and increases the longevity of the restoration[25].

Table II: Summary of the clinical applications of the nanoparticles most commonly used in endodontics.

Applications / NPs		Preserving pulp vitality	Endodontic irrigation	Instrumentation	Intravenous medication	Root canal filling		Pulp regeneration	Restoration materials coronary		
						Cements sealing	GP		RC	CVI	adhesives
AgNP			+++		++	+	+		+	+	+
CS-NP		+	+		+						
G-NP			+		+		+				
MeO-NP (ZnO-NP)		+	+		+	+	+		+	+	+
AuNP			+					+	+		+
BAG-NP		++			+			+			
HA-NP								+	+	+	
Zr-NP									+		+
Other	WS2			+							
	ND		+				+				
	Nano MTA	+						+			
	Nano CaOH2				++						
	Nano CHX		+		+						
	nACP	+							+	+	+
	NZOE					+					
	QPEI					+					
	exosomes							+			

Based on the number of scientific papers published :

(+++): Nanoparticles are used extensively in these fields (++): Nanoparticles are used extensively in these fields (+): Nanoparticles are applied in these fields

CONCLUSION

Scientific and technological advances have opened up new horizons in the field of endodontics, the branch of dentistry that focuses on the treatment of the dental pulp and on the development of new treatments.the surrounding tissue.The application of nanoparticles has emerged as a significant field of study because of their ability to enhance the performance of materials and methods used in endodontics. Because of their extremely small size and unique properties, nanoparticles offer substantial advantages in various aspects of endodontic treatment.Nanoparticles can be used in a variety of endodontic applications, including pulp vitality preservation, root canal irrigation and instrumentation, intracanal medication, definitive root canal filling, pulp regeneration procedures, and coronal filling materials. Nevertheless, the use of these nanoparticles requires an in-depth assessment of the potential risks, in order to understand their defects, their likely cellular impact, their toxicity and their effects on the environment.In addition, it is important to stress that the majority of research into dental nanomaterials is currently limited to in vitro studies. In vivo studies and clinical trials involving patients are still essential to fully assess the efficacy and safety of nanoparticles.Further research is urgently needed to thoroughly assess the long-term effects of nanoparticles in endodontics. This includes an in-depth analysis of their immunogenicity, biocompatibility and/or biodegradability, as well as the identification of potential risks associated with practitioner exposure to these nanoparticles. In addition, it is essential to develop appropriate safety standards to guide their use.

REFERENCES

1. Abbasi E, Milani M, Fekri Aval S et al.

Silver nanoparticles: Synthesismethods, bio-applications and properties.

Crit RevMicrobiol 2016;42:173-80.

2. Abbaszadegan A, Nabavizadeh M, Gholami A et al.

Positively charged imidazolium-based ionic liquid-protected silver nanoparticles: a promising disinfectant in root canal treatment.
Int Endod J 2015;48:790-800.

3. Adini AR, Feldman Y, Cohen SR et al.

Alleviating fatigue and failure of NiTi endodontic files by a coating containing inorganic fullerene-like WS2 nanoparticles.
J Mater Res 2011;26:1234-42.

4. Afkhami F, Forghan P, Gutmann JL, Kishen A.

Silver nanoparticles and their therapeutic applications in endodontics: a narrative review.
Pharmaceutics 2023;15:715.

5. Afkhami F, Rostami G, Batebi S, Bahador A.

Residual antibacterial effects of a mixture of silver nanoparticles/calcium hydroxide and other root canal medicaments against Enterococcus faecalis.
J Dent Sci 2022;17:1260-5.

6. Afrasiabi S, Chiniforush N, Barikani HR, Partoazar A, Goudarzi R. Nanostructures as targeted therapeutics for combating oral bacterial diseases.
Biomedicines 2021;9:1435.

7. Agnihotri SA, Mallikarjuna NN, Aminabhavi TM.

Recent advances on chitosan-based micro- and nanoparticles in drug delivery.
J Controlled Release 2004;100:5-28.

8. Aguiar AS, Guerreiro-Tanomaru JM, Faria G, Leonardo RT, Tanomaru-Filho M.
Antimicrobial activity and ph of calcium hydroxide and zinc oxide nanoparticles intracanal medication and association with chlorhexidine. J Contemp Dent Pract 2015;16:624-9.

9. Ai M, Du Z, Zhu S et al.

Composite resinreinforcedwith silver nanoparticles-laden hydroxyapatite nanowires for dental application.
Dent Mater 2017;33:12-22.

10. Akbari M, Zebarjad SM, Nategh B, Rouhani A.

Effect of nano silica on setting time and physical properties of mineral trioxide aggregate.

J Endod 2013;39:1448-51.

11. **Albrecht C, Scherbart AM, van Berlo D, Braunbarth CM, Schins RP, Scheel J.** Evaluation of cytotoxic effects and oxidative stress with hydroxyapatite dispersions of different physicochemical properties in rat NR8383 cells and primary macrophages. Toxicol Vitro Int J 2009;23:520-30.

12. **Al-Madi EM, Al-Jamie MA, Al-Owaid NM, Almohaimede AA, Al-**

Owid AM.

Antibacterial efficacy of silver diamine fluoride as a root canal irrigant.

Clin Exp Dent Res 2019;5:551-6.

13. **Alves MJ, Grenho L, Lopes C et al.**

Antibacterial effect and biocompatibility of a novel nanostructured ZnO-coated gutta-percha cone for improved endodontic treatment. Mater Sci Eng C Mater Biol Appl 2018;92:840-8.

14. **Alzahrani FM, Katubi KMS, Ali D, Alarifi S.**

Apoptotic and DNA-damaging effects of yttria-stabilized zirconia nanoparticles on human skin epithelial cells.
Int J Nanomedicine 2019;14:7003-16.

15. **Ambalavanan N, Kavitha M, Jayakumar S, Raj A, Nataraj S.** Comparative evaluation of bactericidal effect of silver nanoparticle in combination with Nd-YAG Laser against enterococcus faecalis: an in vitro study.
J Contemp Dent Pract. 2020;21:1141-5.

16. **Anu Mary Ealia S, Saravanakumar MP.**

A review on the classification, characterisation, synthesis of nanoparticles and their application.
IOP Conf Ser Mater Sci Eng 2017;263:032019.

17. **Arif W, Rana NF, Saleem I et al.**

Antibacterial activity of dental composite with ciprofloxacin loaded silver nanoparticles.
Mol Basel Switz 2022;27:7182.

18. **Azaryan E, Hanafi-Bojd MY, Alemzadeh E, Emadian Razavi F, Naseri M.** Effect of PCL/nHAEA nanocomposite to osteo/odontogenic differentiation of dental pulp stem cells.
BMC Oral Health 2022;22:505.

19. **Azaryan E, Mortazavi-Derazkola S, Alemzadeh E et al.**

Effects of hydroxyapatite nanorods prepared through Elaeagnus Angustifolia extract on modulating immunomodulatory/dentin-pulp regeneration genes in DPSCs.
Odontology 2023;111:461-73.

20. Bagga P, Siddiqui HH, Akhtar J, Mahmood T, Zahera M, Khan MS.
Gold nanoparticles conjugated with levofloxacin: for improved antibacterial activity over levofloxacin alone.
Curr Drug Deliv 2017;14:1114-9.

21. Baghdadi I, AbuTarboush BJ, Zaazou A et al.

Investigation of the structure and compressive strength of a bioceramic root canal sealer reinforced with nanomaterials.
J ApplBiomaterFunct Mater 2021;19:1-13.

22. Balsaraf O, Raghavendra SS, Shah D, Sanjyot M, Balsaraf A. Comparative evaluation of antifungal efficacy of conventional endodontic irrigants and chitosan nanoparticles.
J Conserv Dent JCD. 2023;26:226-9.

23. Balto H, Bukhary S, Al-Omran O, BaHammam A, Al-Mutairi B. Combined effect of a mixture of silver nanoparticles and calcium hydroxide against enterococcus faecalis biofilm.
J Endod. 2020;46:1689-94.

24. Bapat RA, Chaubal TV, Dharmadhikari S et al.

Recent advances of gold nanoparticles as biomaterial in dentistry.

Int J Pharm 2020;586:119596.

25. Bapat RA, Chaubal TV, Joshi CP et al.

An overview of application of silver nanoparticles for biomaterials in dentistry.
Mater Sci Eng C Mater Biol Appl 2018;91:881-98.

26. Bapat RA, Yang HJ, Chaubal TV et al.

Review on synthesis, properties and multifarious therapeutic applications of nanostructured zirconia in dentistry.
RSC Adv 2022;12:12773-93.

27. Baras BH, Wang S, Melo MA et al.

Novel bioactive root canal sealer with antibiofilm and remineralization properties.
J Dent 2019;83:67-76.

28. Barros J, Silva MG, Rodrigues MA et al.

Antibacterial, physicochemical and mechanical properties of endodontic sealers containing quaternary ammonium polyethylenimine nanoparticles.
Int Endod J 2014;47:725-34.

29. Baskar K, Saravana Karthikeyan B, Gurucharan I et al.

Eggshell derived nano-hydroxyapatite incorporated carboxymethyl chitosan scaffold for dentine regeneration: A laboratory investigation. Int Endod J 2022;55(1):89-102.

30. Bastos NA, Bitencourt SB, Martins EA, De Souza GM. Review of nano-technology

applications in resin-based restorative materials.
J EsthetRestor Dent 2021;33:567-82.

31. Bellamy C, Shrestha S, Torneck C, Kishen A.

Effects of a bioactive scaffold containing a sustained transforming growth factor-β1-releasing nanoparticle system on the migration and differentiation of stem cells from the apical papilla.
J Endod 2016;42:1385-92.

32. Betancourt J, Cabral-Romero C, Hernandez-Delgadillo R et al. Analysis of the antimicrobial and antibiotic activity of nanoparticles for endodontic use.
Int J Appl Dent Sci 2020;6:85-9.

33. Biz MT, Cucco C, Cavalcanti BN.

Incorporation of AuNP-PLL nanocomplexes in DPSC: a new tool for 3D analysis in pulp regeneration.
Clin Oral Investig 2020;24:1761-7.

34. Bonilla-Represa V, Abalos-Labruzzi C, Herrera-Martinez M, Guerrero-Pérez MO.
Nanomaterials in dentistry: state of the art and future challenges.

Nanomaterials 2020;10(9):1770.

35. Bordea IR, Candrea S, Alexescu GT et al.

Nano-hydroxyapatite use in dentistry: a systematic review.

Drug MetabRev 2020;52:319-32.

36. Cao W, Zhang Y, Wang X et al.

Development of a novel resin-based dental material with dual biocidal modes and sustained release of Ag+ ions based on photocurable core- shell AgBr/cationic polymer nanocomposites.
J Mater Sci Mater Med 2017;28:103.

37. Carpio-Perochena A del, Kishen A, Shrestha A, Bramante CM. Antibacterial properties associated with chitosan nanoparticle treatment on root dentin and 2 types of endodontic sealers.
J Endod 2015;41:1353-8.

38. Chang HH, Tseng YT, Huang SW et al.

Evaluation of carbon dioxide-based urethane acrylate composites for sealers of root canal obturation.
Polymers 2020;12:482.

39. Charannya S, Duraivel D, Padminee K, Poorni S, Nishanthine C, Srinivasan MR.
Comparative evaluation of antimicrobial efficacy of silver nanoparticles and 2% chlorhexidine gluconate when used alone and in combination assessed using agar diffusion method: An in vitro study.

Contemp Clin Dent 2018;9:204-9.

40. Chávez-Andrade GM, Tanomaru-Filho M, Rodrigues EM et al.

Cytotoxicity, genotoxicity and antibacterial activity of poly(vinyl alcohol)-coated silver nanoparticles and farnesol as irrigating solutions.

Arch Oral Biol 2017;84:89-93.

41. Chávez-Andrade GM, Tanomaru-Filho M, Basso Bernardi MI, de Toledo Leonardo R, Faria G, Guerreiro-Tanomaru JM. Antimicrobial and biofilm anti-adhesion activities of silver nanoparticles and farnesol against endodontic microorganisms for possible application in root canal treatment.
Arch Oral Biol 2019;107:104481.

42. Chen J, Zhao Q, Peng J, Yang X, Yu D, Zhao W.

Antibacterial and mechanical properties of reduced graphene-silver nanoparticle nanocomposite modified glass ionomer cements.
J Dent 2020;96:103332.

43. Chung JH, Kim YK, Kim KH et al.

Synthesis, characterization, biocompatibility of hydroxyapatite-natural polymers nanocomposites for dentistry applications.
ArtifCellsNanomedicineBiotechnol 2016;44:277-84.

44. Corral Nunez C, AltamiranoGaete D, Maureira M, Martin J, Covarrubias C.
Nanoparticles of bioactive glass enhance biodentine bioactivity on dental pulp stem cells.
Mater Basel Switz 2021;14:2684.

45. Craciunescu I, Ispas GM, Ciorita A, Leoştean C, Illés E, Turcu RP. Novel magnetic composite materials for dental structure restoration application.
Nanomater Basel Switz 2023;13:1215.

46. Dadkan S, Salari S, Khakbiz M, Atai M.

Mechanical properties of dental adhesives containing gold nano particles.
Proceedings of 5th International Congress on Nanoscience & Nanotechnology.
Nanotechnology (ICNN2014) 22-24 October 2014, Tehran, Iran, 2014.

47. DaSilva L, Finer Y, Friedman S, Basrani B, Kishen A.

Biofilm formation within the interface of bovine root dentin treated with conjugated chitosan and sealer containing chitosan nanoparticles.
J Endod2013;39:249-53.

48. de Almeida J, Cechella BC, Bernardi AV, de Lima Pimenta A, Felippe WT.
Effectiveness of nanoparticle solutions and conventional endodontic irrigants against Enterococcus faecalis biofilm.
Indian J Dent Res 2018;29:347-51.

49. Del Carpio-Perochena A, Bramante CM, Duarte MA, de Moura MR, Aouada FA, Kishen A.
Chelating and antibacterial properties of chitosan nanoparticles on dentin.
Restor Dent Endod2015;40:195-201.

50. Dizaj SM, Lotfipour F, Barzegar-Jalali M, Zarrintan MH, Adibkia K.
Antimicrobial activity of the metals and metal oxide nanoparticles.

Mater Sci Eng C 2014;44:278-84.

51. Dreanca A, Sarosi C, Parvu AE et al.

Systemic and local biocompatibility assessment of graphene composite dental materials in experimental mandibular bone defect.
Materials 2020;13:2511.

52. Elgendy AA, Fayyad DM.

ell viability and apoptotic changes of dental pulp stem cells treated with propolis, chitosan, and their nano counterparts.
Tanta Dent J 2017;14:198.

53. Elkassas D, Arafa A.

The innovative applications of therapeutic nanostructures in dentistry.
NanomedicineNanotechnol Biol Med 2017;13:1543-62.

54. Ertem E, Gutt B, Zuber F et al.

Core-shell silver nanoparticles in endodontic disinfection solutions enable long-term antimicrobial effect on oral biofilms.
ACS Appl Mater Interfaces 2017;9:34762-72.

55. Eshed M, Lellouche J, Matalon S, Gedanken A, Banin E. Sonochemical Coatings of ZnO and CuO nanoparticles inhibit streptococcus mutans biofilm formation on teeth model.
Langmuir 2012;28:12288-95.

56. Eskandari F, Abbaszadegan A, Gholami A, Ghahramani Y.

The antimicrobial efficacy of graphene oxide, double antibiotic paste, and their combination against Enterococcus faecalis in the root canal treatment.
BMC Oral Health 2023;23:20.

57. Franková J, Pivodová V, Vágnerová H, Juráňová J, Ulrichová J. Effects of silver nanoparticles on primary cell cultures of fibroblasts and keratinocytes in a wound-healing model.
J ApplBiomaterFunct Mater 2016;14(2):137-42.

58. Gad MM, Al-Thobity AM, Shahin SY, Alsaqer BT, Ali AA. Inhibitory effect of zirconium oxide nanoparticles on Candida albicans adhesion to repaired polymethyl methacrylate denture bases and interim removable prostheses: A new approach for denture stomatitis prevention.

Int J Nanomedicine 2017;12:5409-19.

59. Galdiero S, Falanga A, Vitiello M, Cantisani M, Marra V, Galdiero M.
Silver nanoparticles as potential antiviral agents.

Molecules 2011;16:8894-918.

60. Ganesh V, Seol D, Gomez-Contreras PC, Keen HL, Shin K, Martin JA.
Exosome-based cell homing and angiogenic differentiation for dental pulp regeneration.
Int J Mol Sci 2022;24:466.

61. Geim AK.

Graphene: Status and prospects.

Science 2009;324:1530-4.

62. Girigoswami K.

Toxicity of metal oxide nanoparticles.

Adv Exp Med Biol 2018;1048:99-122.

63. Gong S, Huang Z, Shi W, Ma B, Tay FR, Zhou B.

In vitro evaluation of antibacterial effect of ah plus incorporated with quaternary ammonium epoxy silicate against enterococcus faecalis.
J Endod 2014;40:1611-5.

64. Gong W, Huang Z, Dong Y et al.

Ionic extraction of a novel nano-sized bioactive glass enhances differentiation and mineralization of human dental pulp cells. J Endod 2014;40:83-8.

65. Guazzo R, Gardin C, Bellin G et al.

Graphene-based nanomaterials for tissue engineering in the dental field.

Nanomater Basel Switz 2018;8:349.

66. Guerreiro-Tanomaru JM, Pereira KF, Nascimento CA, Bernardi MIB, Tanomaru-Filho M.
Use of nanoparticulate zinc oxide as intracanal medication in endodontics: pH and antimicrobial activity.
Acta Odontol Latinoam 2013;26:144-8.

67. Gupta SM, Tripathi M.

An overview of commonly used semiconductor nanoparticles in photocatalysis.

High Energy Chem. 2012;46:1-9.

68. Hajihassani N, Alavi O, Karamshahi M, Marashi SM, Khademi A, Mohammadi N.
Antibacterial effect of nano-chlorhexidine on Enterococcus faecalis biofilm in root canal system: An in vitro study.

Dent Res J 2022;19:80.

69. Halkai KR, Halkai R, Mudda JA, Shivanna V, Rathod V. Antibiofilm efficacy of biosynthesized silver nanoparticles against endodontic-periodontal pathogens: An in vitro study.
J Conserv Dent 2018;21:662-6.

70. Hoveizi E, Naddaf H, Ahmadianfar S, Gutmann JL.

Encapsulation of human endometrial stem cells in chitosan hydrogel containing titanium oxide nanoparticles for dental pulp repair and tissue regeneration in male Wistar rats.
J BiosciBioeng2023;135:331-40.

71. Huang CS, Hsiao CH, Chang YC et al.

A novel endodontic approach in removing smear layer using nano and submicron diamonds with intracanal oscillation irrigation.
Nanomaterials 2023;13:1646.

72. Ioannidis K, Niazi S, Mylonas P, Mannocci F, Deb S.

The synthesis of nano silver-graphene oxide system and its efficacy against endodontic biofilms using a novel tooth model.
Dent Mater 2019;35:1614-29.

73. Jamleh A, Sadr A, Nomura N et al.

Nano-indentation testing of new and fractured nickel-titanium endodontic instruments.
Int Endod J 2012;45:462-8.

74. Jeevanandam J, Barhoum A, Chan YS, Dufresne A, Danquah MK. Review on nanoparticles and nanostructured materials: history, sources, toxicity and regulations.
Beilstein J Nanotechnol 2018;9:1050-74.

75. Joudeh N, Linke D.

Nanoparticle classification, physicochemical properties, characterization, and applications: a comprehensive review for biologists.
J Nanobiotechnology 2022;20:262.

76. Jowkar Z, Hamidi SA, Shafiei F, Ghahramani Y.

The effect of silver, zinc oxide, and titanium dioxide nanoparticles used as final irrigation solutions on the fracture resistance of root-filled teeth. Clin CosmetInvestig Dent. 2020;12:141-8.

77. Karlsson HL, Gustafsson J, Cronholm P, Möller L.

Size-dependent toxicity of metal oxide particles--a comparison between nano- and micrometer size.
ToxicolLett 2009;188:112-8.

78. Khalil R.

Electrodeposition of ZnO in ionic liquid media: physico-chemical studies of the various stages [Thesis].
Sorbonne: Lebanese University Doctoral School ED388, 2018.

79. Khan M, Shaik MR, Khan ST et al.

Enhanced antimicrobial activity of biofunctionalized zirconia nanoparticles.
ACS Omega 2020;5:1987-96.

80. Kim KJ, Sung WS, Suh BK et al.

Antifungal activity and mode of action of silver nano-particles on Candida albicans.
BioMetals 2009;22:235-42.

81. Kishen A, Shrestha A.

Nanoparticles for endodontic disinfection.

Clin Dent Rev 2018;2:11-7.

82. Kumar N, Kumbhat S.

Carbon-Based Nanomaterials. In: Kumar N, Kumbhat S, eds. Essentials in Nanoscience and Nanotechnology.
Hoboken: John Wiley & Sons, 2016. p. 189-236.

83. Kumar R, Umar A, Kumar G, Nalwa HS. Antimicrobial properties of ZnO nanomaterials: A review. Ceram Int 2017;43:3940-61.

84. Kumari N, Sareen S, Verma M et al.

Zirconia-based nanomaterials: recent developments in synthesis and applications.
Nanoscale Adv 2022;4:4210-36.

85. Lai HZ, Chen WY, Wu CY, Chen YC.

Potent antibacterial nanoparticles for pathogenic bacteria.

ACS Appl Mater Interfaces 2015;7:2046-54.

86. Lee DK, Kim SV, Limansubroto AN et al.

Nanodiamond-gutta percha composite biomaterials for root canal therapy.
ACS Nano 2015;9:11490-501.

87. Li Z, Xie K, Yang S, Yu T, Xiao Y, Zhou Y.

Multifunctional Ca-Zn-Si-based micro-nano spheres with anti-infective, anti-inflammatory, and dentin regenerative properties for pulp capping application.
J Mater Chem B 2021;9:8289-99.

88. Liang Z, Chen D, Jiang Y et al.

Multifunctional Lithium-Doped Mesoporous Nanoparticles for Effective Dentin Regeneration

in vivo.
Int J Nanomedicine 2023;18:5309-25.

89. Lin HP, Tu HP, Hsieh YP, Lee BS.

Controlled release of lovastatin from poly(lactic-co-glycolic acid) nanoparticles for direct pulp capping in rat teeth.
Int J Nanomedicine 2017;12:5473-85.

90. Liu C, Tan D, Chen X, Liao J, Wu L.

Research on graphene and its derivatives in oral disease treatment.

Int J Mol Sci 2022;23:4737.

91. Liu S, Zeng TH, Hofmann M et al.

Antibacterial activity of graphite, graphite oxide, graphene oxide, and reduced graphene oxide: membrane and oxidative stress.
ACS Nano 2011;5:6971-80.

92. Loo SC, Moore T, Banik B, Alexis F.

Biomedical applications of hydroxyapatite nanoparticles.

CurrPharmBiotechnol 2010;11:333-42.

93. Luong D, Kesharwani P, Deshmukh R et al.

PEGylated PAMAM dendrimers: Enhancing efficacy and mitigating toxicity for effective anticancer drug and gene delivery.
Acta Biomater 2016;43:14-29.

94. Mandhalkar R, Paul P, Reche A.

Application of nanomaterials in restorative dentistry.

Cureus 2023;15(1):e33779.

95. Martinez-Andrade JM, Avalos-Borja M, Vilchis-Nestor AR, Sanchez-Vargas LO, Castro-Longoria E.
Dual function of EDTA with silver nanoparticles for root canal treatment-A novel modification.
PLoS One 2018;13:e0190866.

96. Mirhosseini F, Amiri M, Daneshkazemi A, Zandi H, Javadi ZS.

Antimicrobial effect of different sizes of nano zinc oxide on oral microorganisms.

Front Dent 2019;16:105-12.

97. Moazami F, Sahebi S, Ahzan S.

Tooth discoloration induced by imidazolium based silver nanoparticles as an intracanal

irrigant.
J Dent Shiraz Iran 2018;19:280-6.

98. Moradpoor H, Safaei M, Mozaffari HR et al.

An overview of recent progress in dental applications of zinc oxide nanoparticles.
RSC Adv 2021;11:21189-206.

99. Moshaverinia A, Ansari S, Movasaghi Z, Billington RW, Darr JA, Rehman IU.
Modification of conventional glass-ionomer cements with N- vinylpyrrolidone containing polyacids, nano-hydroxy and fluoroapatite to improve mechanical properties.
Dent Mater 2008;24:1381-90.

100. Naseri M, Eftekhar L, Gholami F, Atai M, Dianat O.

The effect of calcium hydroxide and nano-calcium hydroxide on microhardness and superficial chemical structure of root canal dentin: An ex vivo study.
J Endod 2019;45:1148-54.

101. Nasim I, Kanth Jaju K, Shamly M, Vishnupriya V, Jabin Z. Effect of nanoparticle based intra-canal medicaments on root dentin micro-hardness.
Bioinformation 2022;18:226-30.

102. Nasim I, Shamly M, Jaju K, Vishnupriya V, Jabin Z. Antioxidant and anti-inflammatory activity of a nanoparticle based intracanal drugs.
Bioinformation 2022;18:450-4.

103. Noronha VT, Paula AJ, Durán G et al.

Silver nanoparticles in dentistry.

Dent Mater 2017;33:1110-26.

104. Obeid MF, El-Batouty KM, Aslam M.

The effect of using nanoparticles in bioactive glass on its antimicrobial properties.
Restor Dent Endod 2021;46:e58.

105. Oncu A, Huang Y, Amasya G, Sevimay FS, Orhan K, Celikten B. Silver nanoparticles in endodontics: recent developments and applications.
Restor Dent Endod 2021;46:e38.

106. Osmond MJ, Krebs MD.

Tunable chitosan-calcium phosphate composites as cell-instructive dental pulp capping agents.
J BiomaterSciPolym Ed 2021;32:1450-65.

107. Özdemir O, Kopac T.

Recent progress on the applications of nanomaterials and nano- characterization techniques in endodontics: A review.
Materials 2022;15:5109.

108. Paiva L, Fidalgo TKS, da Costa LP et al.

Antibacterial properties and compressive strength of new one-step preparation silver nanoparticles in glass ionomer cements (NanoAg- GIC).
J Dent 2018;69:102-9.

109. Pandit S, Gaska K, Kádár R, Mijakovic I. Graphene-based antimicrobial biomedical surfaces. Chemphyschem 2021;22(3):250-63.

110. Parolia A, Kumar H, Ramamurthy S et al.

Effect of propolis nanoparticles against enterococcus faecalis biofilm in the root canal.

Mol Basel Switz 2021;26:715.

111. Pattanaik S, Jena A, Shashirekha G.

In vitro comparative evaluation of antifungal efficacy of three endodontic sealers with and without incorporation of chitosan nanoparticles against Candida albicans.
J Conserv Dent 2019;22:564-7.

112. Pepla E, Besharat LK, Palaia G, Tenore G, Migliau G.

Nano-hydroxyapatite and its applications in preventive, restorative and regenerative dentistry: a review of literature.
Ann Stomatol 2014;5:108-14.

113. Pushpalatha C, Suresh J, Gayathri VS et al.

Zinc oxide nanoparticles: a review on its applications in dentistry.

Front BioengBiotechnol 2022;10:917990.

114. Rabea EI, Badawy ME, Stevens CV, Smagghe G, Steurbaut W. Chitosan as antimicrobial agent: Applications and mode of action. Biomacromolecules 2003;4:1457-65.

115. Raghunath A, Perumal E.

Metal oxide nanoparticles as antimicrobial agents: a promise for the future.
Int J Antimicrob Agents 2017;49:137-52.

116. Rao AC, Venkatesh KV, Nandini V et al.

Evaluating the effect of tideglusib-loaded bioactive glass nanoparticles as a potential dentine regenerative material.
Mater Basel Switz 2022;15:4567.

117. Raura N, Garg A, Arora A, Roma M.

Nanoparticle technology and its implications in endodontics: A review.

BiomaterRes 2020;24(1):21.

118. Rodrigues CT, de Andrade FB, de Vasconcelos LRSM et al. Antibacterial properties of silver nanoparticles as a root canal irrigant against Enterococcus faecalis biofilm and infected dentinal tubules.

Int Endod J 2018;51:901-11.

119. Saghiri MA, Asatourian A, Nguyen EH, Wang S, Sheibani N. Hydrogel arrays and choroidal neovascularization models for evaluation of angiogenic activity of vital pulp therapy biomaterials.
J Endod2018;44:773-9.

120. Semmler-Behnke M, Kreyling WG, Lipka J et al. Biodistribution of 1.4- and 18-nm gold particles in rats. Small 2008;4(12):2108-11.

121. Seung J, Weir MD, Melo MA et al.

A modified resin sealer: physical and antibacterial properties.

J Endod 2018;44:1553-7.

122. Shrestha A, Kishen A.

Antibacterial nanoparticles in endodontics: A review.

J Endod2016;42:1417-26.

123. Singh AA, Makade CS, Krupadam RJ.

Graphene nanoplatelets embedded polymer: An efficient endodontic material for root canal therapy.
Mater Sci Eng C Mater Biol Appl 2021;121:111864.

124. Song W, Ge S.

Application of antimicrobial nanoparticles in dentistry.

Molecules 2019;24:1033.

125. Sreenivasalu PK, Dora CP, Swami R et al.

Nanomaterials in dentistry: Current applications and future scope.

Nanomater Basel Switz 2022;12:1676.

126. Stoor P, Söderling E, Salonen JI.

Antibacterial effects of a bioactive glass paste on oral microorganisms.
Acta Odontol Scand 1998;56:161-5.

127. Tahriri M, Del Monico M, Moghanian A et al.

Graphene and its derivatives: Opportunities and challenges in dentistry.

Mater Sci Eng C Mater Biol Appl 2019;102:171-85.

128. Teymoornezhad K, Alaghehmand H, Daryakenari G, Khafri S, Tabari M.
Evaluating the microshear bond strength and microleakage of flowable composites containing zinc oxide nano-particles.
Electron Physician. 2016;8:3289-95.

129. Thomas SC, Harshita null, Mishra PK, Talegaonkar S.

Ceramic nanoparticles: fabrication methods and applications in drug delivery.
CurrPharm Des 2015;21:6165-88.

130. Tondnevis F, Ketabi MA, Fekrazad R, Sadeghi A, Abolhasani MM. Using chitosan besides nano hydroxyapatite and fluorohydroxyapatite boost dental pulp stem cell proliferation.
J BiomimBiomaterBiomed Eng 2019;42:39-50.

131. Topala F, Nica LM, Boariu M et al.

En-face optical coherence tomography analysis of gold and silver nanoparticles in endodontic irrigating solutions: An in vitro study. ExpTher Med 2021;22:992.

132. Tran DT, Salmon R.

Potential photocarcinogenic effects of nanoparticle sunscreens.

Australas J Dermatol 2011;52(1):1-6.

133. Vasiliu S, Racovita S, Gugoasa IA, Lungan MA, Popa M, Desbrieres J.
The benefits of smart nanoparticles in dental applications.

Int J Mol Sci. 2021;22:2585.

134. Vichery C, Nedelec JM.

Bioactive glass nanoparticles: From synthesis to materials design for biomedical applications. Materials 2016;9:288.

135. Virlan M, Miricescu D, Radulescu R et al.

Organic nanomaterials and their applications in the treatment of oral diseases.
Molecules 2016;21:207.

136. Wang R, Habib E, Zhu XX.

Evaluation of the filler packing structures in dental resin composites: From theory to practice. Dent Mater 2018;34:1014-23.

137. Wang Y, Hua H, Li W, Wang R, Jiang X, Zhu M.

Strong antibacterial dental resin composites containing cellulose nanocrystal/zinc oxide nanohybrids.
J Dent 2019;80:23-9.

138. Wang Z, Zhou Z, Fan J et al.

Hydroxypropylmethylcellulose as a film and hydrogel carrier for ACP nanoprecursors to deliver biomimetic mineralization.
J Nanobiotechnology 2021;19:385.

139. Wong J, Zou T, Lee AH, Zhang C.

The potential translational applications of nanoparticles in endodontics.

Int J Nanomedicine 2021;16:2087-106.

140. Wu D, Fan W, Kishen A, Gutmann JL, Fan B.

Evaluation of the antibacterial efficacy of silver nanoparticles against Enterococcus faecalis biofilm.
J Endod 2014;40:285-90.

141. Xiao S, Liang K, Weir MD et al.

Combining bioactive multifunctional dental composite with PAMAM for root dentin remineralization.

Materials 2017;10:89.

142. Ye M, Shi B.

Zirconia nanoparticles-induced toxic effects in osteoblast-like 3T3-E1 Cells.
NanoscaleResLett 2018;13(1):353.

143. Yin IX, Zhang J, Zhao IS, Mei ML, Li Q, Chu CH.

The antibacterial mechanism of silver nanoparticles and its application in dentistry.
Int J Nanomedicine 2020;15:2555-62.

144. Yousefshahi H, Aminsobhani M, Shokri M, Shahbazi R.

Anti-bacterial properties of calcium hydroxide in combination with silver, copper, zinc oxide or magnesium oxide.
Eur J TranslMyol 2018;28(3):7545.

145. Yudaev P, Chuev V, Klyukin B, Kuskov A, Mezhuev Y, Chistyakov E.
Polymeric dental nanomaterials: Antimicrobial action.

Polymers 2022;14:864.

146. Zakrzewski W, Dobrzyński M, Zawadzka-Knefel A et al.

Nanomaterials application in endodontics.

Materials 2021;14:5296.

147. Zarei M, Javidi M, Gharechahi M, Joybari M., Tajzadeh P, Arefnejad M.
An in vitro evaluation of antimicrobial efficacy of new Nano-zinc Oxide Eugenol (NZOE).
J Dent Mater Tech 2018;7(4):167-73.

148. Zhang X.

Gold nanoparticles: Recent advances in the biomedical applications.

CellBiochemBiophys 2015;72:771-5.

149. Zhang Y, Ali SF, Dervishi E et al.

Cytotoxicity effects of graphene and single-wall carbon nanotubes in neural phaeochromocytoma-derived PC12 cells.
ACS Nano 2010;4(6):3181-6.

150. Zhang Z, Bi F, Guo W.

Research advances on hydrogel-based materials for tissue regeneration and remineralization in teeth. Gels 2023;9:245.

Internet references

151. CultureScience-Chemistry.

Propriétés des nanoparticules d'or [On line]. Available from URL: https://culturesciences.chimie.ens.fr/thematiques/chimie- inorganic/properties-of-nanoparticles-d-
or#:~:text=Les%20propri%C3%A9t%C3%A9s%20physiques%20du%2
0m%C3%A9tal,%2C%20l'or%20devient%20biod%C3%A9gradable.

152. ID glass.

Documentary files Use of a bioactive glass in the

implantable medical devices [Online].

Available from URL: http://www.idverre.net/veille/dostec/coll06- verre-bioactif/coll06-verre-bioactif.php

153. Wikipedia .

Zirconium dioxide [Online].

Available from URL: https://fr.wikipedia.org/wiki/Dioxyde_de_zirconium#:~:text=Le%20dio xyde%20of%20zirconium%2C%20or,is%20a%20solid%20crystalline%20white

154. Wikipedia.

Nanotechnology [Online].

Available from URL:

https://en.wikipedia.org/wiki/Nanotechnology

155. Wikipedia.

Metal oxide [Online].

Available from URL:

https://fr.wikipedia.org/wiki/Oxyde_m%C3%A9tallique

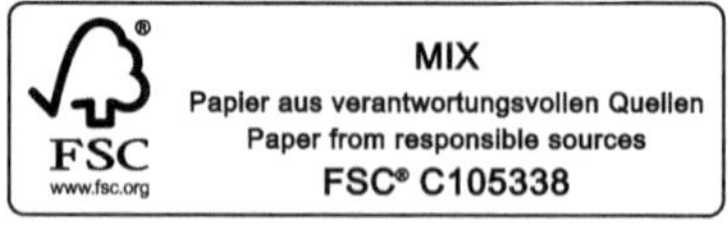

Printed by Books on Demand GmbH, Norderstedt / Germany